Living as Long as I Can
As Well as I Can

James Pomeroy

En Route Books and Media, LLC
St. Louis, MO

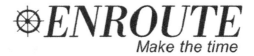

ENROUTE
Make the time

En Route Books and Media, LLC

5705 Rhodes Avenue

St. Louis, MO 63109

Cover credit: Sebastian Mahfood

Copyright © 2022 James Pomeroy

ISBN-13: 978-1-956715-28-6 and 978-1-956715-24-8

Library of Congress Control Number 2022930805

Dedication

This book is dedicated to memories of Don Pomeroy, my dad, John Pomeroy, my twin brother, Donna Fogarty, a cousin, Mitzi Carroll, a pioneer in the care for persons with addiction, and John Bussen, mentor and friend. These five people showed me what living a virtuous life meant.

Contents

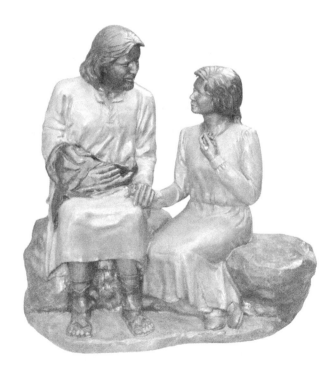

Photo courtesy of CHRISTUS St. Michael Health System.

Preface

The original intent was to describe how the five people identified in the dedication were virtuous living examples. After discussing the project with my family and friends, I decided to broaden the scope by using the experience I had gained in over 40 years of health care experience and my education in health care ministry through the Aquinas Institute of Theology, St. Louis, Missouri. The goal was to produce a book that would be helpful to health care providers, including doctors, nurses, allied health professionals, and chaplains. I also wanted to provide useful information to people who had been diagnosed with a serious illness as well as their families. The aim was to show how one can live well despite the challenges of a medical condition.

I have been fortunate to be able to work with health care professionals within faith-based institutions who honor the dignity and worth of the patients and families they serve. Also, I have been blessed to have been and continue to be cared for by providers who honor life. My experience with cardiologists such as James Hurley and Kevin Hayes in Texarkana, as well as Louis Stickley, Gregory Botteron, Amit Doshi, and Bruce Czarnik in St. Louis, has supported and encouraged me in my active lifestyle. My primary care providers, Dr. Chad Voges in St. Louis and Stephanie

McCorkle, a nurse practitioner in Texarkana, have been equally helpful in my desire to live as well as I can for as long as I can. Their support allows me to approach the topic of living well, despite challenges, with a great deal of confidence.

I have chosen to write a book where each chapter has a specific individual message yet maintained compositional integrity. The goal is to offer the reader information in each chapter that is useful and at the same time provide an entire work that covers the spiritual foundation for living well, individually and collectively.

Finally, I need to acknowledge that this work could not have been completed without my colleagues' assistance in Texarkana; special thanks to Chris Karam, Fr. Lawrence Chellaian, Sr. Jeanne Connell, Francine Francis, and Sue Johnson. They were critical in assuring I had the correct historical information about the hospital. I also thank Bill Brinkmann for reviewing the book's sections that dealt with the Catholic Identity Matrix.

Trudy, my wife, was a great sounding board and critical reader of the manuscript. My niece, Carrie Pomeroy, a teacher and writer, Bob Rothermich, a published author and friend, and my son Jeremy, a Ph.D. scientist and author of several published scientific articles, also reviewed the manuscript. Their insights and suggestions were kind and helpful. Finally, I want to thank Peggy Fagen for diligently proofreading the entire work. Her suggestions were significant in allowing this work to be submitted to the publisher.

I trust that if you are a health care provider or person affected by health care challenges that you will find this book as a valuable reference.

Foreword

This book's basis is my desire to help families and care-givers support those who have life-limiting illnesses. I want to discuss ways, as a friend once remarked, "to live as long as I can for as well as I can."[1] I undertake this task as a person of faith and an experienced business professional who has studied religion and medical ethics. I have negotiated business relationships with Catholic health care organizations and been a Mission Leader in such a facility. I have lost loved ones and faced a life-limiting illness myself, which has shown me that virtuous living can help us live and die with integrity, hope, and peace. I want to share how these principles can help others live that kind of virtuous life, whether caring for others in medical settings or facing life-limiting illness as a patient or family member.

The book is not intended as a philosophical or theological work. I do not doubt that several of my professors would agree that I am not qualified on either topic. It contains both disciples' basics and psychological and social behavioral elements to emphasize particular points I wish to

---

[1] This expression was frequently used by my friend and mentor, John Bussen. John was diagnosed with stage 4 pancreatic cancer in 2014. John continued to live as an example of Christian faith and love for others until his death in August 2015.

make. I utilize the experience I have gained as a health care mission leader and the contributions of colleagues with whom I have had the opportunity to serve over the last 40 years. I must also confess I am a firm believer that living a life of faith prepares us for our glorious transition from mortal to immortal life. Virtuous living allows the "kingdom of God" to begin to be experienced here and now. This book explores our human fascination with death. It deals with living well in the time given to each of us. Finally, it discusses how individuals and organizations can create an environment that allows us to flourish. I emphasize how health care organizations, especially those that proclaim themselves faith-based, can facilitate "living as long and as well as one can."

My niece, Carrie Pomeroy, an accomplished writer in her own right, has suggested that I may have two separate books, which I am trying to fit into this one work. My reply is that I am trying to give the intended audience a book that they can use immediately. I want it to contain information that allows them to make informed decisions. That requires a contextual background concerning the source of faith found in Scripture and access to information concerning the right ways of living.

On the one hand, I want to focus on how we, as individuals, can embrace a life of faith combined with the natural moral law. On the other, I also want to focus on the idea that virtuous living is a corporate (collective) responsibility of all people. In the New Testament, Jesus tells us in Matthew, Mark, and Luke, *You shall love the LORD, your God with all of your heart, with all of your soul, and with all of your mind* (Mt 22:37). The second is like it; *You shall love your neighbor as yourself* (Mt 22:39). Jesus is combining two Old Testament passages, Deuteronomy 6:4-5 and Leviticus 19:9-18, to provide us what is fundamental to correct living. In a like manner, I argue that living a life of virtue is both an individual effort and manifest in our collective action toward each other. I use Catholic health care as an example of how we integrate individual and collective virtuous living to create a community where its members can flourish. Living well cannot be separated from loving others.

For several years, I served in the Vice President of Mission Integration role in a Catholic health care system in Texarkana, USA. CHRISTUS St. Michael Health System has historically been one of the top-performing hospitals in the CHRISTUS Health System. More importantly, it is a hospital with high patient and associate (their term for employees) satisfaction regionally and state-wide, and in 2010 it was named the Best Place to Work in the US for Health Care. It is also an organization that can demonstrate fidelity to its Catholic heritage and identity. In 2018, it was named for the third time as a "Top 100 Hospital" in the nation by IBM Watson Health.™ The study spotlights the US's top-performing hospitals based on a balanced scorecard of clinical, operational, and patient satisfaction data. The system was also one of 13 hospitals to be awarded the Everest Award, an additional honor. The Everest designation honor is for organizations that rate among the top for current performance and rank among the fastest-improving over five years.

Shortly after I assumed the position, the organization chose to be evaluated using an assessment tool called the Catholic Identity Matrix (CIM). Ascension Health developed this assessment tool, and it was refined in cooperation with Veritas Institute, part of St. Thomas University in St. Paul, Minnesota. Bill Brinkmann, one of the original creators of the assessment tool, explains its development in the following way.

> In December 2005, the Ascension Health Sponsor's Council requested that the Ascension Health System office develop a means of assessing the system's Catholic identity. In response to that request, The Ascension Health system office developed the Catholic Identity Matrix, which used the principles of the CHA Shared Statement of Identity (e.g., Promote and Defend Human Dignity, Care for the whole person, etc.) and an organizational maturation framework which tracked the implementation of these principles. The system office conducted a trial assessment in 2006, using a "stoplight (green, yellow, red) assessment process and presented the results to the Sponsors Council. The Spon-

sors approved the CIM framework but requested greater rigor in how the implementation levels were scored and documented. In response to the Sponsor's request for greater rigor, Ascension Health reached out to the Veritas Institute at St Thomas University, which worked extensively on measuring the implementation of organizational principles in a total quality context. Veritas's assessment process for scoring the levels of implementation was integrated into Ascension Health's CIM, and a successful assessment was conducted in 2007.[2]

This decision to submit to the CIM came after a meeting CHRISTUS St. Michael's CEO, Chris Karam, Fr. Lawrence Chellaian, Sr. Jean Connell, and I had with Bishop Anthony Taylor of the Diocese of Arkansas. The Ordinary (Bishop) to whom the organization was responsible was that of the Diocese of Tyler, Texas. Nevertheless, because CHRISTUS St. Michael had begun in Arkansas and continues to have ties to the State (Texarkana is on the border of Texas and Arkansas), it was the practice to continue to meet from time to time with the Bishop of Arkansas. At

---

[2] The information concerning the origin of the Catholic Identity Matrix was provided by Bill Brinkmann, former Vice President at Ascension Health and a collaborator in the development of the Catholic Identity Matrix.

that meeting, our delegation outlined all the essential work and achievements we had produced to demonstrate our identity as a Catholic Church ministry. The Bishop's response, while friendly, did ask a penetrating question: "What makes you a Catholic health care organization?"

What we had emphasized was our "good works" of which any secular organization could boast. The Bishop's question went to the heart of the issue. Why did we exist as a distinct entity if all we did was what any health care organization would do to maintain market share and preserve a nonprofit tax status? The Sisters of Charity of the Incarnate Word had chosen in 1916, despite a strong anti-Catholic sentiment in the community (which, except for a few isolated situations, no longer exists), to come to Texarkana to "extend the healing ministry of Jesus Christ." The Sisters' work over the last 100 years has transformed the city to the point that CHRISTUS St. Michael is seen as the leading example of Christian witness within Northeast Texas. However, in that meeting, we were unable to articulate how accurate our mission statement was.

Following the meeting with Bishop Taylor, the leadership team, in conjunction with the health system leaders of CHRISTUS Health, implemented a plan to assure that we were intentional in our efforts to faithfully continue the mission that our founding Congregation had so heroically begun. The assessment showed exceptional alignment with Catholic health care principles when compared to other

Catholic health care organizations. We were able to demonstrate faithfulness to the "Principles of Catholic Health Care."

These principles include solidarity with the poor, holistic care, participatory workplace, stewardship, respect for life, and acting consistently with the Catholic Church's teachings. What was demonstrated is that by fidelity to the organization's mission statement and values, we were able to materially impact the well-being of the community from the perspective of physical health. The organization has also profoundly affected families with beginning and end-of-life issues. The organization enabled the poor to access care. There is an active effort to demonstrate respect for the dignity of patients, families, and associates of the organization. A stable collaborative relationship with faith leaders in the various religious denominations within the community has also been established. CHRISTUS St. Michael looks to its sponsors as the source of its heritage. The ministry takes pride in assuming the successor's role to the Sisters' charism (a divinely conferred gift of the Holy Spirit).

My predecessor in the position was Sr. Damian Murphy, a Catholic nun from the Congregation of the Sisters of Charity of the Incarnate Word. The Congregation was founded in 1869 and is now based in Houston, Texas. Today, the Sisters have missions in Ireland, Guatemala, El Salvador, Mexico, Kenya, and the United States. They are involved in ministries in health care as part of CHRISTUS

Health System, an international Catholic, faith-based, not-for-profit health system comprised of almost 350 services and facilities, including more than 60 hospitals and long-term care facilities, 175 clinics and outpatient centers, and dozens of other health ministries in Chile, Colombia, Mexico, and the United States. The Congregation also has a vital ministry dedicated to education, social justice, fighting illiteracy and AIDS.

Sr. Damian is a remarkable individual with experience as a nurse, chaplain, administrator, and ethicist. Her work over 20 years at CHRISTUS St. Michael reinforced a foundation established by the Sisters of Charity of the Incarnate Word-Houston Congregation of support for the ministry's mission statement: "To extend the healing ministry of Jesus Christ." Chris Karam, the CEO, fortified Sr. Damian's influence through his model of living. He led the efforts to ensure that our business practices reflected our Catholic health care provider's identity. The commitment to Catholic identity is carried on by a new generation of leaders at CHRISTUS St. Michael. They have all been formed by the Sisters of Charity of the Incarnate Word-Houston Congregation.

I was fortunate to be selected to be the mission leader after Sr. Damian's retirement. My background was much different from Sr. Damian since I had been a Business Development executive with for-profit entities during most of my career. I had worked with many Catholic health care organizations as part of my job. Still, I never had any idea that I would, at some point, be working as a mission leader. My "calling" was made clear to me by Sr. Jean deBlois, a Sister of St. Joseph of Carondolet. Sr. Jean was Director of the Health Care Ministry program sponsored by the Aquinas Institute of Theology in St. Louis, Missouri. For many years, I had a keen interest in scripture study. I had intended to enroll in the Aquinas Institute to study Scripture and theology. Upon seeing my application, Sr. Jean convinced me that I belonged in the health care ministry. I enrolled in the program and spent the next three years having spirited discussions with Sr. Jean that continue even today. I like to tell people that Sr. Jean was the "hardening and tempering process that strengthened me."

Upon graduation, I began looking for opportunities to work in a health care ministry in St. Louis, where I lived. St. Louis is rich in Catholic health care opportunities with Mercy Health, SSM Healthcare, and Ascension Health. Also, the Catholic Healthcare Association maintains its headquarters in St. Louis. I spoke with representatives of each of these organizations but found no corporate office employment opportunity readily available. Brian O'Toole, Sr. Vice President of Mission and Ethics at Mercy Health, did offer sound advice when he suggested that I needed to be "in the trenches." He thought I was best suited for work within a hospital. That advice set me on a course to find a hospital job. After a couple of unsuccessful interviews, I contacted a classmate, Deborah Simmens, who worked for CHRISTUS Health. She informed me of a position in Texarkana and facilitated a telephone interview. They were looking for a mission leader with a strong business background who understood how to integrate "mission and margin." I seemed to fit the bill. So, my wife, Trudy, and I prepared for our new adventure in Texarkana, USA. I was fortunate that the administrative team at CHRISTUS St. Michael was willing to take a chance with a 63-year-old "rookie" mission leader. I was also privileged to have Fr. Lawrence Chellaian as my Spiritual Care Director and "faithful spiritual companion." Fr. Lawrence is an exceptional spiritual leader and confidant.

Our call to discipleship challenged us to leave our past life for an unknown future with an invitation to act as a "servant leader." I am blessed to have a loving spouse who willingly responded to this invitation with me. Trudy's experience solidified our decision to accept this new opportunity during her first visit to Texarkana. As I was being interviewed, Trudy took it upon herself to talk to staff, patients, volunteers, and family members while visiting the hospital. Trudy told me that she "prayed the interviews went well because she felt the presence of Jesus in this place." CHRISTUS St. Michael was where we were blessed to serve!

One additional factor influences me and my view of life as a finite gift. I had several people close to me who lived as well as they could for as long as they could. These were very different people, yet each was strengthened in his or her life experiences by an active faith commitment. I will use my involvement with each of these people to show that the shared experience of faith, especially for those with a life-limiting illness, offers a complete view of "hope."

All too often, we speak of hope as optimism. Optimism is an element of hope, yet it often anticipates an unrealistic expectation for a "miracle" to occur. Unfortunately, for many, faith and hope are based on four faulty assumptions. These assumptions are (1) that faith is more like a social obligation that sets one apart from others, it makes you select; or (2) that faith exists independent of reason, "it just is;" (3) that faith is merely following the rules; if we do what is required, God will take care of us; (4) that all we have to do is trust, and God will make everything go well. Although there is an individual element of truth in all these positions, they fail to consider the internal transformation present in true faith. It is the desire to change one's life from the inside, to repent and undergo a spiritual conversion. This change is called *metanoia,* which means a difference in the way you think and a change of heart. The prophet Ezekiel tells us: *"I will give you a new heart and a new spirit I will put within you. I will remove the heart of stone from your flesh and give you a heart of flesh"* (36:26).

Yet, *metanoia* is not just a private concern that does not require a materially different way of life. Jürgen Moltmann, in his book *Theology of Hope,* understands Christian faith primarily as hope for the future of humankind. In his words, he sees hope as "nothing else than the expectation of those things which faith has believed to have been truly promised by God."[3] As do other contemporary theologians, Moltmann sees God as suffering with humans, offering each of us a better future through the promise fulfilled in Christ's resurrection. His understanding suggests that God can experience suffering. Thomas Weinandy, among others, would argue that God can't suffer, yet he can truly aid us in our pain.[4] My aim is not to refute either position. Instead, for me, the more critical point is, through Christ, we are bound together in faith and hope. This view does not negate suffering but correctly defines pain as a part of the human condition. Hope allows us to endure and, in fact, aids us in living a life of passion for creating a just world. The concept of hope is relevant for how we deal with a life-limiting illness in an era when, all too often, we are being promised cures by modern medicine. These promised cures neither enhance nor improve life quality or allow meaningful interaction with those we love without faith. In the

---

[3] Jürgen Moltmann, *Ethics of Hope* (Minneapolis, MN: Fortress Press, 2012), 20.

[4] Thomas G. Weinandy, *Does God Suffer?* (Notre Dame, IN: Univ. of Notre Dame Press, 2000), vii.

search for a miracle, there is a tendency to enter a conditional relationship with God and fellow humans.

Finally, the reader is free to be critical of my decision to use Christian beliefs to live well. I recognize that there is much to be admired about Eastern as well as the other Abrahamic religions. Our Christian experience is enriched by acknowledging, particularly with the other Abrahamic religions, the existence of one Creator, God. I base my opinion on the following Christian belief. I see God in a descending relationship with humans. *For God so loved the world, that he gave his only begotten Son, that whoever believes in him shall not perish, but have eternal life* (Jn 3:16).

Jesus comes into the world from the Father. He was to experience all that humans experience. God, as demonstrated in Jesus, is not some abstraction or unknowable power. We come to know God in a way that transcends intellectual understanding or knowledge. Knowing allows us to accept and believe that *the Father is in me* (Jn 6:69). It is a response of faith and an acceptance of Christ. I trust that Jesus came primarily to reveal who God is and how we can have a relationship with him. God is one eternal God, but he exists in the relationship of three persons - Father, Son, and Holy Spirit. These three entities exist in one God for all eternity. We tend to think of relationships as being between human beings. Yet, our acceptance of the Trinity shows that relationship is fundamental to knowing God. The Christian relationship with God is one of immanence and transcendence. God is everywhere present. God is manifest in history and the lives of people in both mundane and dramatic ways. God is also transcendent, as the wholly other in the sense that he is unlike his creation. The difference with Christianity is that God became one of us, lived as a human, and made his revelation real in the sense that we experience God in the person of Jesus Christ. Our relationship with God through the mediation of Jesus is ascending as well as descending.

I am convinced that we build a relationship with a personal God upon a foundation of love. It is the approach that will allow each of us to live our lives in a way that will enable the highest degree of freedom. Freedom in the sense I am talking about is the freedom to serve the LORD and our neighbors and to know God through an intimate relationship with Jesus Christ as revealed through Scripture and the Holy Spirit's experience. This understanding of freedom, I am hopeful, will become more apparent as you continue in this book.

Suggested Reading

Unless otherwise noted, scriptural references are taken from the *New American Bible Revised Edition*, the Third Edition. I highly recommend *The Catholic Study Bible*, edited by Donald Senior, John J. Collins, and Mary Ann Getty. The editors provide excellent discussions concerning each of the Books of the Bible. Also, they offer commentary at the beginning of each book, which outlines the writing style and the main points the authors are making.

Introduction

There would soon come a time
when each of us will either be a mystic or a non-believer.
(Fr. Ron Rolheiser quoting Karl Rahner)

Rolheiser used the quote above to express that living a life of faith is more challenging today because the cultural supports that existed in earlier times no longer dominate.[1] Living a life of faith in a secular world requires a deeper understanding of Jesus Christ's message. Throughout this book, I will argue that living a life of faith built around the virtues will lead to happiness that goes beyond mere momentary pleasure and ultimately leads to communion with our Creator.

Death is a part of life and a word with multiple meanings that describes a process that is an account of how one has lived. In the past, like the birth of a person, dying was generally a family, communal, and religious event. How the person would be able to live and relate within the family was of most significant concern. Living was defined by how

---

[1] Ronald Rolheiser, "In Exile," *Saint Louis University Sunday Web Site,* accessed February 20, 2021, https://liturgy.slu.edu/ EpiphanyB010321/reflections_rolheiser.html.

one could contribute to the well-being of the fundamental institutions within which one lived. It is only in relatively recent times that dying has become a medical event principally with the primary goal of extending life at whatever cost. I do not wish to argue about the ethical issues surrounding how "quality of life" is defined. Instead, I want to pay attention to how we can live, which allows us to experience hope consciously. This book is directed at understanding the living process, emphasizing living a virtuous life.

There have been many well-written books on the end of life, which I would strongly encourage you to read. They include the books by Atul Gawande, MD, *Being Mortal,* and Angelo E. Volandes, MD, *The Conversation.* These are thought-provoking and insightful books about the end-of-life and treatment, primarily in the United States. Both writers challenge existing ideas and practices as well as offer suggestions for change. Both use real-life examples in their discussions of how we can humanize end-of-life care. They also discuss ways to reimagine elder care to allow people to have purpose and meaning as they mature. It is a discussion that emphasizes valuing the wisdom and experience that comes with age. They talk about maintaining the dignity of all people with particular emphasis on older people. Additionally, Dr. Jeffrey Long and Paul Perry in *God and the Afterlife* present a strong case that the descriptions of those who have had a near-death experience provide evidence of a life hereafter. More importantly, they acknowledge an omnipresent God "who radiates incredible love, grace, and acceptance."[2]

I also draw upon Ernest Becker's book, *The Denial of Death*, which won the Pulitzer Prize in 1974. Reviewers call it a brilliant and passionate answer to the "why" of human existence. Becker, a philosopher, describes the ultimate existential question- man's refusal to acknowledge his mortality. In doing so, he sheds new light on humanity's nature and issues a call to life and its living that still resonates.

Finally, I intend to directly focus on spirituality as a driving force in our lives. For me, spirituality is focused on God, as revealed in Scripture. I plan to show that through faith, we can come to grips with the inevitability of death. Moreover, through faith, we can learn to live, as Matthew Kelly says in his book, *The Four Signs of a Dynamic Catholic,* in a way that allows us to be the "best versions of ourselves."[3] The idea of being the best version of ourselves is not confined to Christians alone; it is something, in faith, that each of us should strive toward daily.

---

[2] Jeffrey Long and Paul Perry, *God and the Afterlife: The Groundbreaking New Evidence for God and near-Death Experience* (New York, NY, NY: HarperOne, an imprint of HarperCollins Publishers, 2017), 3.

[3] Matthew Kelly, *The Four Signs of a Dynamic Catholic* (Hebron, KY: Dynamic Catholic Institute, 2012), 185.

I have adopted a view focusing on living a virtuous life, individually and corporately, as a way of enabling us to "live as well as I can, as long as I can." I support this contention by looking at various cultures, finally using the Christian view of virtue as a moral way of living. I discuss how virtue ethics is not merely a particular way of acting but applies to corporate responsibility. I then use my experience with a Catholic health care provider to demonstrate how an organization can influence its associates and create an environment that encourages communities to flourish. At the end of each chapter, I have identified writing that has influenced my thinking. Offered then is a summary of each chapter.

Chapter One is entitled, Why Do We Fear Death? We have difficulty trying to harmonize an all-powerful God who teaches love and mercy and yet allows suffering and pain to exist. To deal with the paradox, we develop all types of explanations that often border on superstition or transactional relations with God rather than faith. We begin to see modern medicine as the purveyor of miracles. A setting is being created in which providers are reluctant or fearful of how the information they provide will be used. They do not want to be sued or seen as withdrawing hope. We lose the message of Christ's gift of salvation in viewing a relationship with Jesus as an if/then proposition.

The Judeo-Christian view is not the only faith tradition that deals with mortality. I contrast the relation of humans to the gods of other practices for comparison purposes. Where others have either a hostile or a distant relation with supernatural powers, the Judeo-Christian God created a desire for order in the world. God, and most especially Jesus and the Holy Spirit in Christianity, have an interactive relationship. God wants humans to have happiness and provides the way to happiness through virtuous living.

Chapter Two is an examination of how one views one's mortality. The chapter briefly discusses the human desire to have a meaning or legacy assigned to their lives. It also deliberates on how humans attempt to defer or avoid thinking about their mortality. Finally, the chapter identifies similarities and differences in how humanity interprets immortality.

Chapter Three is written explicitly as a reference from the Old and New Testaments for direct caregivers, spiritual care providers, family, and those persons who have a life-limiting illness. I write more extensively about the Old Testament because its teaching is often either not known or misinterpreted. It deals with ideas gleaned from Jewish Scripture as foreshadowing the Christian perspective, as this is the viewpoint from which I arrive at my belief. The chapter primarily uses Jewish Scripture within the religious and philosophical context. They were written to establish that belief in a power beyond human capability and frailty is reasonable. The chapter discusses how humanity works to address the question of how meaning in life is determined. It then considers expectations for a life hereafter. Attention is paid to how we can use Biblical interpretation tools to understand how God's message concerning salvation is conveyed through language and writing styles. Biblical passages from both Old and New Testaments are examined to demonstrate a rich tradition of thinking about the afterlife. God's saving power is revealed within the writings.

Chapter Four begins with assessing the Mediterranean culture's influence on Christian and Jewish beliefs and traditions about the afterlife. While the Middle-Eastern idea influenced Judaism, its offshoot, Christianity, adds Greek, Roman, and Egyptian ideas to its practice and beliefs. These ideas are central to how mortal and immortal life are viewed from the Christian perspective.

The final portion of the chapter deals with St. Paul's teaching on the centrality of the suffering on the cross, death, and resurrection in terms of salvation. Paul's teaching reveals that the kingdom of God is available through faith in Jesus Christ. Humanity's freedom from sin and damnation is a result of Christ's redemptive action. It is a message of hope that has stood the test of time.

Chapter Five deals with the often confusing and misunderstood topic of miracles. Throughout the writing, I have made the point that Jesus' message of salvation, His life of right living, death, and resurrection are central to the mission to reveal God to the world. Nevertheless, it is an emphasis on Jesus' miracles that provides the attraction for all too many. I have called this a transactional or "if/then" relationship that relies on faith that is conditional.

I have located miracles as signs of God's presence in the world in the person of Jesus Christ. My view of miracles is built on the foundation of faith. It is our faith that allows us to endure and have hope. Hope, as I describe it, is coming to know God's love and mercy. C.S. Lewis describes two types of miracles: those of Old Creation and New Creation.[4] Miracles of New Creation offer us the promise of a new state of being. They point to our ultimate destiny, completing the human journey to be in full communion with God. St. Thomas Aquinas terms this as the *beatific vision*.[5]

Most of our prayers are for what Lewis terms miracles of Old Creation. That is, we petition for supernatural intervention in our human world. Such prayers fall into five broad groups. We ask for temporary or time-specific suspension of natural law; we seek physical healing; we plead to have power over death; we seek relief from emotional pain; we ask that our daily needs be supplied. All of these petitions seem to come from a sense of one's powerlessness.

---

[4] C. S. Lewis, *Miracles: A Preliminary Study* (San Francisco: HarperOne, 2001), 215, 233.

[5] Thomas Aquinas, "Question 23. How the Passions Differ from One Another," *Summa Theologiae: I answer that* (Prima Secundae Partis, Q. 23), 2017, http://www.newadvent.org/ summa/2023.htm.

They are often made when we have exhausted all our human efforts. I conclude the chapter with a question: Do miracles still occur? I define the essential features of a miracle and then give my answer to the question.

Up to this point, I talk about the human longing to understand what will become of us after our mortal life is complete. I have also discussed how we can see God's power as either a payoff within a transactional relationship or a way to reach the *beatific vision*.

Chapter Six deals with how one can live in such a way to prepare for the kingdom of God. I have referred to Cardinal John Henry Newman's concept of how humans deal with death. He teaches that we can have notional assent in which death is put out of mind. On the other hand, in real assent, I acknowledge my relationship with others, most importantly, to God. I recognize my sinfulness and that it is through the grace of God that I am offered salvation.

I contend that we can realize true freedom through living in a manner consistent with the cardinal and theological virtues. Freedom is defined in the Catholic Church's Catechism as "the power rooted in reason and will, to act or not to act" (*CCC* 1731). Freedom attains its highest perfection when it is directed toward God. Freedom is that which draws one closer to God. I conclude the chapter with examples of holy people who intentionally elected to live virtuous lives.

Chapter Seven deals with the issue of autonomy and informed consent as an obligation for all people. The section also discusses the current medical community's attitude and practices regarding life-limiting illness. It provides specific guidance in addressing issues that arise with those experiencing chronic illness. I include an extended discussion concerning palliative care's appropriateness to serve as a means for adding longevity and demonstrating a belief in the dignity of and love for one's neighbor. It is caring that honors the desire to live as long as one can, as well as one can.

Chapter Eight delves into the question of how to live a life in service and love. It discusses the concept of how faith-based organizations can influence a community. I begin with a brief overview of the foundational story of the Sisters of Charity of the Incarnate Word-Houston Congregation, leading to their ministry in Texarkana. Their story is similar to many of the women's religious congregations' health care ministry formation. I then discuss how the transition to lay leadership has affected the perception of health care ministries. I discuss the significance of health care ministries to ask the question, "Who do they say we are?" I also discuss why it is essential for those seeking care to be aware of the perspective that the health care organization embraces. Is sufficient attention given to its identity as a faith-based, Catholic health care provider? The question to ask is whether the provider is committed to its mission, and how is that commitment manifest? That has led many to engage in an audit to determine their fidelity to the ministry's legacy, mission statement, and values.

The final chapter will provide concrete (but not exhaustive) examples of how CHRISTUS St. Michael Health System has worked to create a culture of dignity, compassion, and empowerment as a means to that end. The chapter will show how one organization, being attentive to its mission and the community (including its associates), can have a profound corporate influence and serve as a model for others. Examples of how fidelity to Catholic health care principles is evident in the ministry will be offered.

I conclude with my thoughts concerning the challenges facing faith-based health care in a secular society. Health care organizations must take the same approach to evaluate their ministry's fidelity to their mission statement and proclaimed values related to their clinical and business practices. Assuring commitment to the mission and intentionality in continuous improvement of performance requires that organizations either develop or take advantage of existing discernment tools. Ministries cannot simply proclaim but must demonstrate that they perform and that their practices have a measurable impact.

Suggested Reading

Being Mortal, Medicine and What Matters in the End, by Atul Gawande, MD, is an easy-to-read discussion concerning how modern medicine can improve the quality of life and deal more effectively with the inevitability of death. While the book only deals with spirituality issues in a limited manner, it demonstrates that care for the other, as expressed in Jesus' command in chapter 15 of John's Gospel, is to love one another.

The Conversation, by Angelo Volandes, MD, deals with many of the end-of-life issues addressed by Dr. Atul. He adds a significant contribution in focusing on the necessity to have honest conversations with those being served by the medical profession. Informed consent is a topic I will discuss at length later in this book.

Chapter One

Why Do We Fear Death?

Now I lay me down to sleep,
I pray the LORD my soul to keep,
And if I die before I wake,
I pray the LORD, my soul to take.

I would say this prayer as a youth as it was taught to me by my mother. This prayer seems very frightening as I look back. I likely would have had many sleepless nights had I put much thought into what I was saying. I had a recent experience with death that was illustrative of how we deal with the fragility of life at a young age. My grandson was given a gerbil as a gift to celebrate his first communion. Ike lived in a specially designed cage, which gave him room to roam and a clean, safe place to sleep. He had no predators and a caregiver who was generous and loving. Ike died after three years. His death was predictable as the average life expectancy of a gerbil is 3-4 years. Nevertheless, Alex, at that time a ten-year-old, immediately broke into tears; Mason, 8 years old, showed compassion by his immediate concern for Alex's well-being. Landon, the 5-year-old, said now, "Ike was with great-grandpa," who had recently died.

The common denominator was that the boys had not contemplated Ike's death. Yet, their responses were very personal expressions of how they experienced the event. Some weeks removed from the occurrence, the response of each child was also different. Mason and Landon had largely moved on; Alex decided he did not want to replace Ike. His decision reminds me of a similar event in my life at about the same age as Alex.

My twin brother and I regularly walked about a half-mile to cross a busy street to catch a bus to go to the local YMCA for swimming lessons. Our dog Soupy often followed us to the bus stop and then ran home after we were safely on the bus. One day, as Soupy began to go home, a car hit him. I immediately ran home. I arrived crying and screaming, "He's dead; he's dead!" My parents ran with me to the bus stop. Upon arrival, my mother discovered I was talking about the dog and expressed with obvious relief, "It's only the damn dog." She had thought I was talking about my brother. We never had another pet. My brother and I both agreed we never wanted to deal with such an event ever again.

Years later, my twin brother died as a result of choking on a piece of meat. I was angry that his life could end in such a "crazy" way. He was 33 years old and just offered a job as a Vice President at a major food company. He had two daughters, the apple of his eye, and a wife who was the love of his life. How could this happen? My response was to retreat into an isolated existence for nearly 8 years. I was active in my job and church, but I did not enter any real friendships. The fear of losing another person close to me was something I dealt with by my denial of relationships. Each of us deals with the overhang of the inevitability of death in ways that protect us from fear about what happens when we die.

Fortunately for me, John Bussen, one of the influences for this book I spoke of earlier, recognized my isolation and invited me to join a group of men who met at 6:30 AM on Saturday mornings to share their faith. We were young men who needed to finish our meeting to coach and attend our kids' various athletic events. We have continued to meet for over 30 years. For me, it was John and the others who were the presence of Jesus that changed my life. These events were and have become part of the process of my living, which has been transformative. My fear of death put me on the road to isolation. My friend's invitation offered me the promise of hope and set the foundation for my life's journey to discover how to be a servant-leader at the CHRISTUS St. Michal Health System.

After I had worked at CHRISTUS St. Michael for about one year, a friend asked me what surprised me most about working in a hospital. This person knew that I had been involved as an administrator or business development professional in health care for nearly thirty-five years. My answer shocked him. I told him, "That people die in hospitals." Most of us think of hospitals as places of healing, and they are. Nevertheless, in today's world, hospitals also serve as places where we deal with the most chronic diseases-simply, the sickest of sick people. People that before the middle of the 20th century would not have survived. The ability to deal with disease processes that would have been fatal in the past is a tremendous achievement. I have experienced such advances myself having had by-pass surgery and an implanted cardioverter defibrillator (ICD). These medical advances have allowed me to continue to live a full and rich life for the last 20+ years.

Hospitals are also places where the process of dying can be interrupted for extended periods. Our ability to achieve what would have been impossible only a few decades ago now allows people like me to live full and meaningful lives. It is a remarkable achievement. Yet, these same medical and technical advances have created an expectation that miracles are routine. Any unwillingness on the part of caregivers to "do everything" signifies the caregiver's lack of faith, a giving up of hope. In many instances, it is considered an issue of equity of care. Patients and families sometimes claim there is a withholding of care due to payer status, race, gender, sexual orientation, or socioeconomic position. The idea that "anything is possible" creates an expectation that the choice to discontinue nonbeneficial care (note, I do not use the term "futile" care) is subjective and discriminatory. Hospitals that I have worked with never stop providing care; rather, they redirect care to benefit the patient. No one is futile since we can provide care that is appropriate to the situation. Care does not need to be restorative to be beneficial.

I want to clarify that the parties were sincere in their concern in the situations in which I have been involved. It is more accurate to say that they experienced the dissonance C.S. Lewis discussed in his book, *The Problem of Pain*. It seems people cannot harmonize the idea of an all-powerful God allowing suffering. Lewis allows that all creatures experience pain. Yet humans have a unique quality:

> In the most complex of all creatures, Man (humans), yet another quality appears, which we call reason. He is enabled to foresee his own pain, which henceforth is preceded by acute mental suffering, to foresee his own death while keenly desiring permanence.[1]

Humans can anticipate pain and suffering. As a result, many of us spend enormous energy and time trying to avoid or deny the eventuality of suffering in our lives.

In her groundbreaking book, *On Death and Dying*, Elisabeth Kübler-Ross labeled this initial phase of coming to grips with our mortality as a denial. In denial, the patient,

---

[1] C. S. Lewis, *The Problem of Pain* (London: HarperCollins, 2002), 2.

family, and frequently the caregiver embark on a quest to solve the problem. Another test, another opinion, another treatment, a miracle drug, and ultimately divine intervention if enough "prayer warriors" can be enrolled. Kübler-Ross maintains that, like many defense mechanisms, denial can provide some temporary benefit. She says, "denial can serve as a buffer after unexpected, shocking news, allows the patient to collect himself and with time mobilize other, less radical defenses."[2] Unfortunately, all too frequently, we see unrealistic expectations support the denial phase. What do I mean?

Look at medical advertising. How often do we see well-known health care systems using carefully crafted messages to imply they can do what no other organization can? If you pay attention to advertising, you will find claims to curing everything from erectile dysfunction to obesity, late-stage cancer, and heart failure. Just listen to the messages without mentioning the increasingly high costs for these "miracle" drugs or deductibles and co-pays for hospitalization. You will come away believing anything is possible. It is all about preserving life--no matter how compromised the patient or unhealthy the lifestyle. The expectation of a miracle is implied by institutions aimed at cancer care. The ubiquitous nature of specialized cancer treatment hospitals or special-

---

[2] Elisabeth Kubler-Ross, *Death and Dying* (New York: Macmillan, 1969), 39.

ized programs within a larger institution brings attention to this dreaded disease and creates consumer demand for the service. There can be no doubt that advertising of these services has increased awareness and stimulated the early detection of breast and other forms of cancer. It is even likely that competition for the consumer dollar has encouraged advances in treatment that would not otherwise have been possible. The downside of increased competition for the health care dollar has all too often led to the illusion that all cancer can be "defeated." I use the term illusion because credible service providers would never categorically state that they can cure without qualification. The message receiver, looking for any sign of relief, often hears the illusion, not the fact.

Direct-to-consumer advertising of pharmaceuticals is pervasive in print and television advertising. Drug companies are estimated to spend better than $20 billion per year in advertising to physicians. Direct to consumer (primarily television, print, or radio) advertising is estimated at another $5.2 billion.[3] Health care organizations use billboards, TV, radio, and print advertising to convince you that they

---

[3] Christina Sarich, "Pharma Companies Spend 19x More on Marketing than Research, and Returns Are Dropping," *Natural Society*, May 02, 2017, accessed December 14, 2018, http://naturalsociety.com/research-development-new-drugs-not-paying-off-6321

are better than the competitors. It is truly an aggressive approach by organizations that use compassion and concern for the patient as the "beard" to increase market share and facilitate horizontal and vertical growth. My opinion is not a sweeping indictment of health care systems, which can provide valuable service to the communities they serve. Instead, it begs the question we need to ask: is this an illness or health care system we are promoting? If we are concerned about health, our focus is on lifestyle, economic empowerment, justice (fair opportunities), access to preventive services, and outreach to marginalized communities. The recent evidence of Covid-19's dramatic effect in minority communities points to the need to focus on health.

If we follow the money, we can see the payout in terms of insurance reimbursement; Medicare and Medicaid are centered on illness care. The ability to influence a hospital or physician to use certain drugs is an essential motivator for spending. Therefore, the ability to reassure the caregiver or patient that any medical condition, no matter how advanced, can be improved at a minimum and cured as the promise is critical to sustain and grow the health care industry. We know from all the talk about the Patient Protection and Affordable Care Act (ObamaCare) that health care already accounts for 18% of the economy. This fact makes health care a big business! The combination of patients and families seeking the ultimate cure and health care providers needing to protect and even expand market share leads to an environment in which the ability to meet any expectations is implied. These proposed outcomes are given along with the appropriate disclaimers. At one time or another, you have asked yourself, "Why would I take this drug or undergo treatment after hearing all the disclaimers?" The ad tells us that the condition for which we are concerned improves for the vast majority and then reports all the side effects in small print (or fast talk). The point is, these ads are not to educate or warn; they are to cultivate the need for their particular product or service.

Caregivers are placed in situations that are often "no-win." They take the path of the least resistance in testing and undertaking procedures that frequently have no beneficial effect. The good news is that for most patients, including me, technological advances and new medical discoveries have allowed American medicine to deal effectively with illness and disease in ways that could not have been imagined 100 years ago. Nevertheless, a growing number of people, due to age or a chronic, life-limiting illness, will not benefit from aggressive, curative treatment. Fortunately, as we learn more about dealing with patients with persistent, life-limiting diseases, there has been remarkable growth in palliative care. For these patients, hope and faith are two critical yet misunderstood concepts that I will discuss later.

It is not only the medical industry that makes claims of the miracles being routine. I recently traveled on a portion of Interstate 70 near the St. Louis International Airport when I saw a billboard that proclaimed, "GOD CAN CURE CANCER." A local evangelical ministry placed it there. While its claim is hard to argue, it made a remedy seem to be as simple as joining this ministry. All too often, we humans like to make promises for God. Dietrich Bonhoeffer, a German theologian whom the Nazis killed during World War II for allegedly being part of a plot to kill Hitler, saw God as not a *deus ex machina* who saves us in time of need. Bonhoeffer said, "God is for the world only by stepping back from it and in this way giving it time and opportunity to be itself."[4]

The idea of God's miraculous intervention is a component of the four false assumptions I discussed earlier in this work. Bonhoeffer believed such a request of religious faith was exploitive, taking advantage of human weakness and ignorance. Bonhoeffer spoke of God as an entity to which we come to know: *God saw all that he had made, and behold, it was very good* (Gn 1:31). Bonhoeffer did not want to deny the reality of life and its inevitabilities. Our relationship with God should not be dependent on a "delivering up" when all else has failed and the natural consequences of a situation begin to emerge.

---

[4] Marcia Pally, "Theological Resistance," *Commonweal Magazine*, February 14, 2021. https://commonwealmagazine.org/theological-resistance.

As I noted earlier, I have been part of a small group of men who meet each Saturday morning to study Scripture and share our ideas. We have met for over 30 years. During that time, we have matured from actively playing soccer and softball, being competitive runners, and even fielding a couple of triathletes as active seniors, to no longer being competitive athletes. In our time, we have had three members with major heart surgery, three with prostate cancer, various orthopedic chronic conditions, a stroke, and one member die of pancreatic cancer. Thankfully, he could avail himself and his family of supportive and compassionate palliative and hospice care services.

We have spent a good deal of time considering our mortality. Hope and faith have been the main topics of discussion as we progress from a secular view of those two terms to a more theological and spiritual vision. We have come to realize that, like those whom Jesus healed, we are all mortal even though each of us has experienced incredible new medical knowledge and technology. We recognize the rest of the stories from the scriptures of the person cured of leprosy, the little girl raised from her death bed, and all the other stories that each of them eventually died. Death is an eventuality for each of us; our faith and hope allow us to live well. So, let's talk about faith and hope from the perspective of living well.

My pastor, Fr. Bob Burkemper, leads an adult scripture study that focuses on Jesus' ministry. In Mark's first chapter, he noted that Jesus could cure a person of demons or Peter's mother-in-law of fever or even a man with leprosy. These stories also appear in chapters 7 and 8 of Matthew and chapter 4 of Luke. What is peculiar to Mark 1:34 is the writer declares: *And he healed **many** who were sick of various diseases and cast out many demons.* This language in Matthew and Luke is raised to a new level when the writers of those books use the same pericope (a coherent selection or extract of an author's writing):

> *When it was evening, they brought him many who were possessed by demons, and he drove out the spirits by a word and cured all the sick.* (Mt 8:16)

> *At sunset, all who had people sick with various diseases brought them to him. He laid his hands on **each** of them and cured them.* (Lk 4:40)

Why is it important to point out that Mark states that Jesus healed many, and Matthew and Luke believe it is crucial to assign unrestrained power to Jesus' healing? Mark's version of the healing stories includes the element of faith as being essential. Matthew and Luke appear to show Jesus' power is in His ability to heal "all." The Gospel writers were evangelists first, and as such, Matthew and Luke were emphasizing power. Both Mark and Luke tell us that Jesus proclaimed His purpose as proclaiming the good news, *for that is why I was sent* (Mk 1:38; Lk 4:43). When we focus solely on the supernatural power of Jesus, we miss the real point of his ministry. Mark does not feel compelled to say Jesus heals all because it is not central to the mission of Jesus' message of repentance and faith. Commentators on Mark refer to Jesus' reluctance to build His ministry on miracles as the "messianic secret."

William Wrede, a German New Testament scholar who was born in Hanover and worked as a professor at Breslau, has argued (although with a good deal of dissent from other scholars) in his book *Messianic Secret in the Gospels* (1901) that Jesus' instruction to keep quiet about His work in Mark 1:43-44 is an effort to conceal His divinity.

And he sternly charges him, and sent him away at once, and said to him, "see that nothing you say to anyone, but go and show yourself to the priest, and offer for your cleansing what Moses commanded for a proof to the people.

Wrede observed that in Mark's narrative Jesus was concerned that if He were to reveal in any way His sense of self-understanding about being the Messiah, those around him would have expected such to have been expressed in a way consistent with contemporary understanding of a Davidic

Messiah, warrior leader, and King.[5] Jesus' ministry is, however, founded on mercy and compassion. Jesus' healing pericopes all demonstrate his love. He did not come as a conqueror or miracle worker in the conventional sense; instead, he offered salvation through suffering and service. The 1st-century Mediterranean world interpreted illness and disease as being associated with the person's demons or sinfulness (or His family). The ability to cure one of illnesses was then considered something that must spring from a power higher than its demons or sinfulness. Jesus' miracle stories are a way to demonstrate to the people of that time that His power comes from His divinity. Yet, if people recognized him solely based on healing and miracles, then He was fully aware that His message of repentance and faith would be lost. Miracles prefigure the decisive messianic miracle, which is the cross and the resurrection. They are acts of healing that foreshadow the greatest act of healing.

Fr. Burkemper made a thought-provoking observation while discussing the synoptic gospels' healing stories. He remarked that "faith, based on signs, is doubt looking for proof." If our faith is dependent on a transactional relationship with Jesus, then it is not faith at all, but doubt that says, "Show me you have the power." It is a challenge to God as opposed to trusting in God. A transactional relationship is

---

[5] William Wrede, *The Messianic Secret* (Cambridge: J. Clarke, 1971), 41.

based on an if/then proposition; it is not a faith relationship. That is, it is dependent on a social contract or agreement. For instance, if I pray for Susan to be healed and faithfully attend church, then Jesus will heal Susan. My actions are not based on faith; instead, they are dependent on an implied result (contractual obligation) that is expected of Jesus, part of the transaction. We often see this in times of trouble or illness. We hope to enter a bargain with God. There is an expectation of a tangible reward if we are willing to do something we believe has value to God. This transactional relationship with Jesus is another example of one of the four wrong ideas about faith: we "trust" that we will be taken care of because we profess our Christianity. Our status as Christians provides us with armor against evil without any requirement made for us to act. It suggests that by merely declaring the label "Christian," I am protected no matter how I behave. I have heard the expression, "He/she is a Christian; how can God let this happen?"

Luke's Gospel is forthright in preaching that faith is not a passive activity, but one in which the Christian is in a dynamic relationship with Jesus Christ and one's neighbors. Luke's Gospel (along with Mark's) calls his readers to action and has among its themes conversion, transformation, and a response of faith. This transformation was termed *metanoia* previously. It is the acceptance of the prophetic message of Jesus, which begins at the start of his public ministry (Lk 4:16-30). He identifies that he is the fulfillment

of the prophecies. It is an active engagement with Jesus'
message to turn one's life. It is a message that calls for repentance.

Faith then is a combination of obedient attention to the
hearing of the Word and endurance. Luke Timothy Johnson, citing Lk 8:15 and 17:5-6, calls faith "a commitment of
the heart that can grow and mature."[6] An essential element
in response to faith is the commitment to prayer as an example of how one relates to Jesus Christ. Thus, if we are to
use Luke's Gospel as a guide, we see that faith and conversion are actions that demand that people change their behavior. Christians, rather than just trusting that "everything
will be all right if we only "trust," are required to serve others and to share with those in need. Being a Christian is an
active and engaged process of faith in Christ's message and
its use to interact with the world. For Luke, the *kingdom of
God is among you* (Lk 17:21). For Christians, this means
that the arrival of the kingdom begins with conversion. It is
the faithful's deeds as imitators of Christ that provide a view
of the kingdom of God. The kingdom of God for Luke is an
internalized transformation manifested in our outward
demonstration of charity toward others. To be a disciple
means being transformed by God's Word, thus becoming a
living example of the conduct fitting to the Gospel message.

----

[6] Luke Timothy Johnson, *The Gospel of Luke.* Edited by Daniel J. Harrington. (Collegeville, MN: Liturgical Press, 2006), 24.

Luke's Gospel message is one of charity. It is built upon the notion that Deuteronomy 6:5 and Leviticus 19:18 should be read as one single commandment. Thus, loving one's neighbor has the same strength as loving God. It is located within the Gospel just before the Good Samaritan story, which I will discuss later as fundamental to Catholic health care and how we treat others. Jesus' reply to the law-yer in the story is central to how we live individually and collectively.

Summary

Within the chapter, I have pointed out our near-obsession with identifying some medical cure for virtually any type of malady, be it physical or emotional. We invest an inordinate percentage of our resources in seeking medical miracles. Often, as a last resort, we seek to bargain with God. This transactional relationship is conditional and not reflective of true faith. Seeking to identify ways to alleviate physical and emotional suffering is a laudable goal yet incomplete without the commitment to a life built around the model which Jesus Christ has offered.

Suggested Reading

The Problem of Pain by C.S. Lewis, a writer well known for his Narnia series of books, is a readable explanation from the author's Christian perspective. It describes what divine love is, what pain is, why humans can feel pain, and a divine purpose to suffering.

On Death and Dying by Elisabeth Kübler-Ross gives the now-famous five stages of death: denial and isolation, anger, bargaining, depression, and acceptance. For many health care professionals and families experiencing end-of-life with a loved one, it has become an essential way for them to explain what is occurring.

Chapter Two

The Desire to Live Forever

For the wages of sin is death,
But the gift of God is eternal life
In Jesus Christ our LORD. (Romans 6:23)

I am a big fan of the "old-time" radio. On a recent short drive, I turned on a science fiction story about humans in some distant future who had achieved immortality. They attained this goal by eliminating all illnesses and other factors (war, natural catastrophes, etc.) that reduced longevity. This situation seemed idyllic at the onset, yet as the story progressed, it was clear that immortality was not all that great. First, the persons in control soon recognized they had to extinguish human desire and ambition from those who came after them to maintain their power. New life was discouraged, as no one was dying. Scientific knowledge was a closely held secret among those in control. The people were to be appeased by the ability to go without want or fear (especially death). The problem arose when a small group of "mutants" was found with a defect, which caused them to retain a desire to have meaning in their lives. They wanted

31

to accomplish something, to have meaningful relationships. This small group ignited a revolt that ultimately resulted in those in control being overthrown. Human passion was allowed to emerge again. The end of the program had death being reintroduced to this world. Some could see this result as a punishment. I would argue that it demonstrates human life's natural desire to have a purpose and meaningful relationships. Immortality, when seen isolated from faith, has implications. The story highlights our fascination with prolonging life. It also opens our eyes to the unexpected consequences that accompany a temporal vision of immortality-- that is, a life without purpose and meaning.

Where do we go? What happens after we die fascinated and puzzled people throughout history. Some of our most ancient encounters with our forebears are through artifacts that portray the transition of death. The earliest oral traditions, sagas, and myths speak of the journey beyond our body's door. There is even a concept called Terror Management Theory (TMT) that is brought on by the awareness of the self's inevitable death. TMT was first described in 1986 by social psychologists Jeff Greenberg, Tom Pyszczynski, and Sheldon Solomon based upon Ernest Becker's ideas. In their book, *The Worm at the Core: On the Role of Death in Life*, the authors report that when Becker was near death, he is said to have told Sam Keen, a philosopher, as the latter was interviewing him in his hospital as he was dying of cancer, "You are catching me in *extremis*. This event is a test of everything I've written about death. And now I've got a chance to show how one dies... how one accepts his death."[1]

TMT tells us that humans share a biological bias toward self-preservation in the service of reproduction with all life forms. We are unique in our capacity for symbolic thought, which fosters self-awareness and the ability to reflect on the past and ponder the future. This ability spawns the realization that death is inevitable and can occur at any time for reasons that cannot be anticipated or controlled.[2] The awareness of death led humans to create ways to explain how we are created. It also led them to seek ways to assure immortality, either literally or in the sense of leaving a legacy. We try to show that both forms of immortality are possible. We perpetuate this idea by maintaining cultural beliefs that provide a sense that life is meaningful by offering an account of the universe's origin. We create prescriptions for appropriate behavior and assurance of immortality for those who follow cultural dictates. Immortality is afforded to souls, heaven with an afterlife, and reincarnations, in one form or another, occur in all major religions. This view of humans suggests a world in which we must construct sto-

---

[1] Sheldon Solomon, Jeff Greenberg, and Thomas A. Pyszczynski, *The Worm at the Core: On the Role of Death in Life* (London: Penguin Books, 2016), vii.

[2] Ibid.

ries that allow us to avoid the confrontation of the reality of
death. We achieve this result through scenarios that offer us
an afterlife rich in rewards for a life well-lived or a punishment for one not so well-lived. The determination to live
well is often based upon the prescriptions outlined in some
form of religious principles. Remarkably, these spiritual
principles often have considerable variation yet provide a
foundation of faith for which the adherent can find comfort.

Ernest Becker, in his book, *The Denial of Death*, states
that:

> In other words, the fear of death must be present be-
> hind all our normal functioning in order for the organ-
> ism to be armed toward self-preservation. But the fear
> of death cannot be present constantly in one's mental
> functioning, or else the organism could not function.[3]

His point is that the ability to deal with the ever-present
biological certainty of death is too much for us to endure.
Therefore, as Becker explains, we create paradigms that either have humans who deny or ignore their fate or are overly sensitive to their mortality. He says:

---

[3] Ernest Becker, *The Denial of Death* (New York: Free Press
Paperbacks, 1997), 16.

On the one hand, we see a human animal who is partly dead to the world, who is most "dignified" when he shows a certain obliviousness to his fate when he allows himself to be driven through life: who is most "free" when he lives in a secure dependency on powers around him, when he least in possession of himself. On the other hand, we get the image of a human animal who is overly sensitive to the world, who cannot shut it out, who is thrown back on his own meager powers, and who seems least free to move or act, least in possession of himself and most undignified.[4]

I would agree that both ways of looking at life, as Becker describes, can lead to a dismal picture of human existence. I would also maintain that each view provides a foundation for humans to successfully deal with what many writers have termed "man's existential dilemma." An existential dilemma is not the moment in which I question the very foundations of my life: whether this life has any meaning, purpose, or value? Instead, it is the ability to appreciate the consequences of our actions and dread the unknown. We have a consciousness that we are both intuitive animals and rational beings capable of anticipating the future. This future includes fear or at least intermittent anxiety about our mortality. Sr. Jean deBlois, in a workshop with physicians at

---

[4] Ibid, 24.

CHRISTUS St. Michael Health Center in 2015, addressed this reluctance to face the fact of death when she cautioned the doctors for using terms like "the patient passed away" when informing families of the death of a patient. She asked, "Why are we afraid to use the word death or died? She suggested that it is our fears that restrict our ability to be forthright in discussing death. Animals have a comfortable ignorance defined by their instincts alone; humans have the burden of anticipating and predicting (correctly or not) the future. As such, we know that ultimately, we will all die. This understanding of our final destiny creates what Becker and others term the "final terror" of self-consciousness.[5] This combined intellectual and emotional experience has led humans to consider death as an inevitable state of being and create myths to support that understanding.

Ancient Myths that Provide Context for Fear of Death

In pursuit of understanding the meaning of life and our place in that picture, humans have developed stories that provide a rationale for death. That rationale is often framed as a punishment due to humans disordering the relationship with divine powers. This disordering can come in disobedience, assumptions of power, and desire for knowledge not authorized. Often, it is a combination of these desires

---

[5] Ibid, 70.

that causes the divine powers to limit humans and other creatures to mortal lives. With the certainty of death, divine authority can, and in the case of the monotheistic and Eastern religions, offer humans an opportunity for immortality to reward a life well-lived.

I shall briefly discuss well-known, ancient Middle Eastern, non-Judeo-Christian explanations of how humans are subject to a finite life dominated by the whims of a detached god(s). In them, death appears as a punishment controlled by the gods. Moreover, humans are seen as created to serve the gods. Later in this work, I will offer an alternative view that maintains death's reality, not as a punishment, but as an opportunity to reach a sense of completeness for each person.

1. The myth of Adapa is the Mesopotamian story of the Fall of Man. It explains why human beings are mortal. Ea, God of wisdom, creates the first man, Adapa, and endows him with immense intelligence and wisdom but not immortality. When the great God Anu offers immortality to Adapa, Ea tricks Adapa into refusing the gift.

2. In the myth of Baal, according to folklore, Yam, the sea god, demanded that Baal be his slave. He sent messengers to Baal, asking him to surrender, but Baal attacked the messengers and drove them away. Baal then fought with Yam and, using two magic

weapons, defeated him and seized the water's control. In the story, Yam represents water's destructive nature: rivers and seas flood the land, ruin crops, and kill animals. Baal represents water's positive powers: rain and dew, providing the moisture needed to grow crops. After conquering Yam, Baal complained that he had no house like the other gods did. El agreed to let the crafts god Kothar build Baal a beautiful home. When it was finished, Baal held a great feast, but he did not invite Mot, god of death and the Underworld, or send him respectful presents. Intensely insulted, Mot asked Baal to come to the underworld to dine. Although afraid, Baal could not refuse the invitation. The food served at Mot's table was mud, the food of death, and when Baal ate it, he was trapped in the underworld.

3. The myth of Gilgamesh is a Babylonian myth that tells the story of woe among great god-men heroes who challenge the gods themselves for the earth's rule. When Gilgamesh's friend Enkidu is killed, he searches for the key to immortality by finding the great flood hero, Utnapishtim. Gilgamesh fails the test of immortality but has a second chance when given the plant of continued rejuvenation. He loses the plant to a serpent and must return home fully mortal and relegated to living with his lot.

These stories are offered here to demonstrate that humans have an enduring desire to explain how we came to be. The accounts describe our relationship with powers beyond our human abilities. In Genesis, the act of forming humanity is the high point of God's creativity. The entire creation account in Genesis 1 leads up to the creation of humans. God has created an environment in which humans can live. Besides, time has been designed to allow for how humans can govern their lives. The claim *God created mankind in His image; in the image of God, he created them; male and female, he created them* (Gn 1:27) expresses the worth of human beings as this description of creation is only used for humans. Gerhard Von Rad explains that the Hebrew word used for image is *selem,* which has various interpretations, including physical resemblance and humanity's spiritual dimension. Von Rad says, "The whole man is created in God's image."[6] Some have suggested that humans are both body and soul, which is a distinctly Greek notion. It is more likely that the "image of God" refers to the command to have dominion over the earth as God's representative. Pauline Viviano notes that humans are significant because they have a special relationship with God as the connection between creation, creatures, and God.

---

[6] Gerhard Von Rad, *Genesis. A Commentary.* (Translation by John H. Marks.) Revised Edition, trans. John H. P., (London: SCM Press, 1972), 55-56.

"As God is the ruler of the heavenly realm, so humanity, as God's representative, is the ruler of the earthly realm."[7] This interpretation of humanity's role vis-à-vis God is entirely different from the Near-East myths' contentious relationship.

The authors of Genesis 1 did not invent the creation story. It follows an order similar to an ancient Babylonian creation myth, the Enuma Elish (also known as The Seven Tablets of Creation). The story, one of the oldest in the world, concerns the birth of gods, the universe's creation, and human beings. In the beginning, there was only undifferentiated water swirling in chaos. The creation narrative comparison between this story and Genesis 1 is striking. Foster McCurley explains that:

> Statements about creation from a faith perspective attempt to evaluate that which has come into being and to understand its role in the order of things. Whether a person of faith views creation negatively (as in Hinduism) or positively (as in the Bible), the issue at stake is

---

[7] Pauline A. Viviano, *Genesis* (Collegeville, MN: Liturgical Press, 1985), 12-13.

the relationship of the created life to whatever caused its origins and other created things.[8]

McCurley pointed out that the relationship between the gods in the Near East is often one of the humans acting as slaves. The link within the Abrahamic traditions is one of God working in concert with humans, creating them as a perfect image. In Genesis 1:26-27, the writer has God saying:

Then God said: 'Let us make human beings in our own image, after our likeness. Let them have dominion over the fish of the seas, the birds of the air, and the tame animals, and all the creatures that crawl on the earth, and over the wild animals and all the creatures that crawl on the ground.' God created mankind in His image; in the image of God, he created them; male and female, he created them.

This image of humans stands in direct contrast to how the creation of stories in the ancient Near East portrays their gods' relationship. This bond between humans and God depicted in Genesis reaches its zenith with the Incarnation of Jesus.

---

[8] Foster R. McCurley, *Proclamation Commentaries: The Old Testament Witnesses for Preaching* (Philadelphia: Fortress Press, 1978), 9.

The Judeo-Christian story of creation demonstrates God's orderly plan of creation with its purpose of providing a paradise for humans to flourish. The Genesis story is in stark contrast to the other myths that have been described. In the Genesis narrative, God creates a perfect world for the benefit of humans. It is a well-ordered world that only requires obedience to God's will that they not eat of the tree in the Garden's center. Cardinal Joseph Ratzinger, who became Pope Benedict XVI, tells us:

> The Garden is an image of the world, which to humankind is not a wilderness, a danger, or a threat, but a home that shelters, nourishes, and sustains. It is an expression for a world that bears the imprint of the Spirit, for a world that came into existence in accordance with the will of the Creator.[9]

Unlike the other ancient narratives, the Genesis story shows God being present from the beginning, making God the Creator of everything. God provides humans with the gift of creation. Humans are asked to build upon and keep it for the purposes for which it was created. Ratzinger states

---

[9] Joseph Ratzinger, *In the Beginning...A Catholic Understanding of the Story of Creation and the Fall*, trans. Boniface Ramsey (Grand Rapids, MI: William B Eerdmans Publishing Company, 1995).

that "we see that the world, which was created to be one with its LORD, is not a threat but a gift and a sign of the saving and unifying goodness of God."[10] This view contrasts with the competition and conflict seen between humans and the gods in the other creation narratives described.

At the time of the creation story's writing, it is believed there is a considerable risk that the Israelites would give in to the seductive promises of Eastern fertility cults. Ratzinger observes that these cults' temptation was the possibility of extending human existence beyond the limits set for it by God at creation.[11] These temptations led to doubting the covenant and the community's fidelity to that covenant. The result is the development of a disordered relationship with God. Doubt about the promise invites people to look for ways to free themselves from their existence's supposed limitations.[12] Ratzinger identifies two variations for the ways that humans seek to "free" themselves. He describes them as aesthetic and technical effects to eliminate the limitations of existence. Ratzinger describes aesthetic effects as reducing morality to that which is "artistic incompetence." Good and moral are no longer important— only competence counts. Thus, what we can do is what we

---

[10] Ibid, 65.

[11] Ibid, 82.

[12] Ibid, 68.

may do.[13] The second variation identified is the technical effect. The question asked is, what can we do without regard to what we should do? In other words, we strip out good and moral issues and focus only on the potential to accomplish. I have often discussed with doctors the difference between doing to or for a patient. Modern medicine can do many remarkable technical procedures that save and enrich life. Physicians are often placed in a situation where they are asked to or believe they must provide procedures to patients for which there is no reasonable hope of benefit and may create harm. The moral question is stripped out of the equation when we do because we can, without limitation.

Both the aesthetic and technical ways of eliminating the limitations of humans' existence represent a worldly pursuit of good that leads us to live as though God either does not exist or is only necessary when we have no other alternative. By that statement, I have seen patients, families, and providers depend on promises of miracles made in advertising (disregarding all the side effect warnings), suggesting we can overcome all. Only when the reality of such promises' ineffectiveness is made clear do we turn to God.

My approach to discussing the Genesis story was not to describe the account as factually accurate as it sets out creation conditions. Instead, I rely on the teaching and the

---

[13] Ibid.

thinking of the best, most reliable Scripture scholars. They describe these stories as symbolic narratives that communicate divinely inspired truths. As divinely inspired, they are not purely myth as we generally define the term as "a made-up" story. I look at the Genesis creation narrative as a Christian trained in the Catholic tradition of scholarship that recognizes the Bible as written by humans using literary forms common to humans. These writers have the Holy Spirit's influence in helping them to reveal God's truth. These stories are not untrue, vaguely reliable, or childish but rather show a profound understanding of how the origin of creation and humankind is communicated.

In his 1995 book, "*In the Beginning ...: A Catholic Understanding of the Story of Creation and the Fall,* Ratzinger writes: "It has become clear that the biblical creation narratives represent another way of speaking about reality than that with which we are familiar from physics and biology."[14] I believe he is clarifying that the story of creation and the "original sin," which resulted from Adam and Eve's eating from the tree, is a symbolic way for humans to understand God's ways. Chapters 1 and 2 of the Book of Genesis describe the perfect creation of the world. Chapter 3 tells us how humans lost their immortality, which culminates in our dread of death. In Chapter 4, we find jealousy and murder. How could this happen? Chapter 3 allows the writ-

---

[14] Ibid, 13.

er to offer us the reason that humans are now condemned to death. In his article, "The Fall-A Second Look: A Literary Analysis of Genesis 2:4-3:24," Dennis Bratcher provides us with a contextual perspective to view the creation/fall story.

The first creation narrative is God-centered. The second narrative's concern is more human-centered. In Genesis 2, God is depicted as creating humans before the rest of the creatures, indicating that creation is incomplete without humanity. In this account, the man is created first, and then the rest of the animals are produced for human's sake. Humans are at the heart of creation. Bratcher comments that in Chapter 2:7:

> The close relationship between the man and his world is emphasized by the similarity of two Hebrew words: the man (Hebrew, *adam*) was created from the ground (Hebrew, *adamah*). "Ground" and "dust" (v. 7) serve to emphasize the fragility of humanity and the total dependence of the creature on the creator. In this story, humanity possesses no inherent immortality, no spark of the divine that removes him from His earthly existence. The man is simply given breath by God, something which he shares with animals. Some older translations use the word soul in this verse. The Hebrew word *(nephesh)* has a wide range of meanings, but here simply means "person" (as NIV, RSV). There is no sense of the later Greek and Christian ideas of body, soul, and

Spirit. Such conceptual categories are alien to Hebrew thinking and complicate the passage with ideas not related to the story. The point is simply that this dust does not live and cannot live until God gives it breath. Breath, life itself, is a gift from God.[15]

In the second creation story, it quickly becomes apparent that humanity is the concern of this story. In this account, the man is created first, and the world is then created for him; he is at the heart of creation. This ordering underscores the commission given to humanity to be responsible for all that God has created. Creation is inherently good as *God looks at everything he had made, and he found it good* (Gn 1:31). These verses affirm the dignity and worth of this frail human creature. Humans have a special place in creation because God has prepared the world as a place where they can live. This faith affirmation about the place of humanity in God's creation is sustained throughout the biblical traditions. The issue the story is subtly developing involves what humanity does in God's world.

A traditional reading of these first chapters of Genesis gives us a framework for showing God's creation and how humans are involved in it. It serves the purpose of setting

---

[15] Dennis Bratcher, "The 'Fall' - A Second Look A Literary Analysis of Genesis 2:4-3:24," accessed January 18, 2020, http://www.crivoice.org/gen3.html.

the stage for all human history's relationship with God. Bratcher tells us:

> It is a story about who God is, who we are as human beings in God's world, how we respond to God, and how God responds to us. It is a story about the human condition. Ultimately, it is a story about us. It is a story that confronts us with who we are in relation to God. If we listen carefully, if we allow ourselves to be caught up into the story, we begin to see ourselves standing before the forbidden tree, torn between obedience to God and our freedom to choose our own way. [16]

Humans are given considerable latitude, but it is limited. God determines the order of the world and establishes the boundaries. The prohibition from eating the fruit of the tree in the middle of the Garden symbolizes boundaries. The defining feature here is that God has heretofore demonstrated loving care for humanity. It is the moral refusal of humans to obey God that justifies God's imposition of mortality. The concept of suffering and pain are also introduced in Genesis 3:17-19.

> *To the man, he said: Because you listened to your wife and ate from the tree of about which I have commanded*

---

[16] Ibid.

you, You shall not eat from it, Cursed be the ground be-
cause of you! In toil shall you eat its yield all the days of
your life. Thorns and thistles, shall it bring bear for, and
you shall eat of the grass of the field. By the sweat of your
brow, you shall eat bread until you return to the ground
from which you were taken: From dust you are dust, and
top dust you shall return.

Adam and Eve's desire to have complete freedom results in the couple's ordered, harmonious world disintegrat-
ing. The world now becomes a place of alienation and chaos. They immediately became aware of their nakedness.
Their shame and guilt cause them to try to hide from God.
The couple finds that they have lost the capacity to relate to
God in the way they did before. God decreed they could not
be allowed to take fruit from the tree of life and live forever.
There it was; human disobedience separated them from living forever.

Robert Miller makes an interesting observation concerning the Tree of Life. He speculates that God banished
Adam and Eve from Eden after eating from the Tree of
Knowledge of Good and Evil; *they would now experience*
pain, toil, and inequality between man and woman (Gn
3:16-18). Eating from the Tree of Knowledge of Good and
Evil ended the special relationship that God had with humans through *Blowing into his nostrils the breath of life, and*
the man became a living being (Gn 2:7). The perfect rela-

tionship between God and humans had been disrupted by the act of eating from a forbidden tree. A merciful God did not want Adam and Eve to eat from the Tree of Life, which would have condemned them to a life of toil, pain, and inequality that was a fate worse than death.[17] Thus, in this way of thinking, Eden's banishment was a sign of God's mercy and love.

It was not God who caused this turn of events--it was Adam and Eve who chose not to live in God's world on the terms established by God. It must be noted that God does not impose an immediate death penalty upon the couple. They are given the gift of life, a second chance, albeit outside the Garden. In this act, God shows profound mercy and grace. This grace, as we know, becomes manifest in the person of Jesus Christ. God demonstrates His intense love for humanity despite their disobedience. While physical immortality is removed, the idea of a "second" chance is provided. God and humans' relationship is one in which love and mercy are always made available by God. Bratcher offers a good summary when he writes:

> From this story, we learn that God chooses to exercise his sovereignty for the good of His creation and for humanity. God simply chooses to offer forgiveness ra-

---

[17] Robert D. Miller, *Understanding the Old Testament: Course Guidebook* (Chantilly, VA: The Great Courses, 2019), 24.

ther than impose what His own law requires. God is not "just" in this story, at least not by any external standard of legal justice. This willingness of God to be "unjust" in order to reclaim His creation is the definition of grace. God's merciful "unjustice" both allowed the couple to live and covered their guilt. This "unjustice," this grace remains the only hope that any sons of Adam and daughters of Eve have.[18]

The interpretations of the Biblical creation stories presented show that understanding those narratives shows how God is revealed to us. It is a model that does not try to "factualize" the creation stories. Instead, the purpose is to reveal God's mercy and love, as demonstrated in action toward humanity in their disobedience. The modern understanding of the Bible came about partly because of discoveries in astronomy, geology, and biology. There were also developments in hermeneutics (the science and art of Bible interpretation). Hermeneutics gives us an outline for understanding the Bible. The framework revolves around four keywords: observation, interpretation, evaluation, and application. The keys are at the heart of all approaches to finding out what the Bible means. They provide the structure of what questions you ask of the text and when.

---

[18] Bratcher.

- Observation: What are the basic facts of the passage, such as the meaning of all the words?
- Interpretation: What did the author mean in its historical setting?
- Evaluation: What does this passage mean in today's culture?
- Application: How can I apply what I have learned to how I live my life?

Interpretation then means we must first discover what the passage meant in the author's day and age. Then we must find its message for us in today's culture. Observation and interpretation apply to the first step; evaluation and application refer to the second. The techniques of hermeneutics allow the Genesis account of creation (Gn 1:1-31, 2:1-3) to be analyzed as follows:

- Observation: The creation story is similar to other ancient creation stories but modified to stress that there is only one God, an all-powerful God, who lovingly created the universe and everything in it, including men and women.
- Interpretation: The writers intended to confirm that God was the creator of all and that creation was not from something. Creation was fashioned by an uncaused First Cause greater than itself. Time, space, and the universe have not always existed, but God

has ever existed, and God's existence is the cause for the presence of all else that exists.

- Evaluation: From the first chapter of Genesis to the last episode of revelation, the Bible tells of one true God who created everything and loves all His creation.

- Application: We can examine our own lives to see if we are putting God above worldly concerns such as today's "false gods" and "idols" of wealth, status, power, success.

The story of Creation is then not a scientific description. It is a way that humans try to understand the mystery of how we came to be and, importantly, why we are mortal. As noted earlier, this effort to understand how we came to be and what will become of us when our temporal lives end is a universal question. Jason Boyette, in *12 Major World Religions: The Beliefs, Rituals, and Traditions of Humanity's Most Influential Faiths,* describes how Hindus, Buddhists, Muslims, representative of the world's other great religions, ask the same questions.[19] A brief description of those beliefs and practices gives us a fuller appreciation of the human desire to understand creation.

---

[19] Jason Boyett, *12 Major World Religions: The Beliefs, Rituals, and Traditions of Humanity's Most Influential Faiths* (Berkeley, CA: Zephyros Press, 2016), 8.

The Muslim story of creation is consistent with the Judeo-Christian narrative of events. Thus, observationally, it is compatible with the religions that share an Abrahamic tradition. It varies in interpretation. Muslims believe that the present life is a trial in preparation for the next realm of existence. When Muslims die, they are washed and wrapped in a clean, white cloth (usually by a family member) and buried after a special prayer, preferably the same day. Muslims consider this a final service that they can do for their relatives and an opportunity to remember that their existence here on earth is brief. The Islamic view of salvation is quite different from the Christians' idea of grace and salvation being gratuitous (unearned and unearnable) gifts of God. The penalty for sin in Islam is death, and it is recognized that everyone sins. The individual must pray for forgiveness but has no assurance of heaven in the afterlife and must work hard to earn God's favor.[20]

One of the best-known Vedic creation myths in the Hindu tradition relates to the sacrifice of Purusha, the primal man from whose body the universe was created. The gods cut up Purusha, took the quarter of him that was manifest in their realm, and placed it upon the sacrificial fire. The Vedic deities Indra, Agni, and Vayu, were born from

---

[20] John D. Morris, "Do Muslims Believe in Creation?" *The Institute for Creation Research*, December 10, 1992, online at https://www.icr.org/article/do-muslims-believe-creation/

this action, together with the cardinal points of the universe: animals, humans, and the four varnas (orders). For the Hindu, humanity is caste into a cycle of repetitive incarnation samsara. Samsara is the continuous cycle of life, death, and reincarnation, which is driven by karma. Karma is the principle of cause and effect, which has actions in a past life affecting one in the present. Life is seen as a continuous series of burdensome and often painful experiences. Through breaking the cycle of karma through individual spiritual development, a reverence for all life forms, and a person's sacrifice, one places oneself in a position to be released from the cycle of life and death.

The Buddhist tradition holds that creation is inconceivable since it has no beginning or end. The Buddhist interest is not so much in what got us here as it is in what we do about it now. The Buddha often refused to answer questions concerning the world's origins because it did not lead to liberation from suffering (*dukkha*).[21] Rather than use terms such as stress or pain, *dukkha* is defined as the first of the Four Noble Truths that teaches all human experience is fundamentally transient and mundane and interferes with the ability to attain Nirvana due to the clinging to "rites, desires, and things."

The Four Noble Truths are: life is suffering, suffering has a cause, craving and attachment can be overcome, the

---

[21] Boyett, 128.

path toward the cessation of craving and attachment is the Eightfold Path.[22] The Eightfold Path includes the right understanding, purpose, speech, conduct, livelihood, effort, alertness, and concentration. Craving for and clinging to impermanent states and things produces karma, which leads us to be caught in an endless cycle of death and rebirth. Humans' tendency can be overcome by seeing the universe as impermanent and illusionary (right understanding). One then can follow by renouncing all attachment to desires through the selfless perspective. Nirvana is achieved when the craving for impermanent states and things is extinguished.[23]

The Buddhist creation story does not contain a beginning, as do other creation stories. It assumes a cosmos ends, and new ones begin. I summarize the Buddhist creation myth in some detail. It is a precise model of a narrative that attempts to explain how evil was introduced into the world through humans' attachment to material things. These creation stories help us to understand not only how we came to be; they describe how suffering is allowed.

---

[22] Ibid.

[23] Ibid, 123.

Summary

This chapter has been directed at addressing the human desire for immortality. Great attention has been paid to how humans have endeavored to make sense of a relationship with God using both Abrahamic and Eastern belief systems to demonstrate how that question is answered. It is a conversation that started in a shared understanding of a relationship with God or gods. It seeks to explain, as people unified by faith, to describe a bond with an immanent and transcendent entity. It is a metaphysical discussion in that it is an effort to make sense of the ultimate cause and constituent elements of reality. While these creation stories are not objectively verifiable, they contain a reality constructed by objective and subjective reality. That is, they provide the elements of what we believe. The Abrahamic creation stories are an essential object of faith that God has revealed. The ultimate purpose of faith is some form of enlightenment. For the Christian, that means through the mediating power of Jesus. The act of faith involves trust in something or someone, for the Christian that is Jesus Christ. Second, the act of faith is how we live our lives. It includes intellectual acceptance, which is formalized in propositions, practices, and creeds. The act of faith is voluntary; that is, it is a conscious decision. Finally, faith is an inner sense of who we are.

Coulter-Harris establishes that immortality, especially involving the soul, is a "shared teaching of Hinduism, Judaism, Buddhism, Christianity, Islam, and native and tribal religions" throughout the world.[24] This belief has resulted from the human desire to seek answers to why we become sick and die. What becomes of us after our physical being becomes no more than the substance from which we were created? The conclusion is that humans have a spirit or soul that gives them purpose, which allows them to live a life with meaning. Moreover, that soul lives on after death and provides us with the hope of experiencing the *beatific vision*. This state of being is a state in which we are in complete union with God. Thomas Aquinas reasoned that we could only be entirely happy when we are in full unity with God. Such harmony is more profound than anything we can imagine or even understand through contemplative prayer. For many, it is only available through the direct perception of God enjoyed by those in heaven. We may experience what many call "God moments" in which we have an extraordinary, mediated experience of God's presence (miracles, for instance). On the other hand, the beatific vision is direct and immediate knowledge of God's presence only available in heaven.

---

[24] Deborah M. Coulter-Harris, *Chasing Immortality in World Religions* (Jefferson, North Carolina: McFarland & Company, Inc., 2016), 142.

Over the next few chapters, I will endeavor to discuss how God's Word, for the Christian, provides us with what the Old and New Testament consider afterlife and emphasizes the subject of hopefulness. There is a recurring theme of confidence, which argues that humans can overcome sin. We are capable of repentance despite Augustine's influential teaching that Original Sin makes human moral behavior nearly impossible. If it were not for the gift of the Grace of God, humans could not behave morally. I contend that it is God's gift of grace that allows humans to choose to live a virtuous life freely, thereby allowing one to live "as long as I can as well as I can," to quote my friend John Bussen. This approach is designed to harmonize the cardinal virtues with the theological virtues to live a life that serves God's will.

Selected Reading

12 Major World Religions: The Beliefs, Rituals, and Traditions of Humanity's Most Influential Faiths, by Jason Boyett, is a comprehensive, easy-to-understand exploration of the 12 major world religions presented in an unbiased fashion. The author looks at creation narratives and the ideas about the afterlife that these faith traditions embrace.

Chapter Three

Thoughts from Scripture

"Even though I walk through the valley
of the shadow of death,
I will fear no evil, for you are with me;
your rod and Your staff comfort me." (Psalms 23:4)

I believe it is essential for those experiencing a life-limiting illness and those providing care within a faith-based perspective to be familiar with how Judeo-Christian scripture views the hope of humans. We are often troubled when faced with questions concerning mortality because we lack a fundamental understanding of what scripture tells us concerning life and the hope for a complete relationship with God. I have often heard physicians, nurses, and other caregivers express regret at "not having the right words" to comfort patients seeking guidance. We turn to chaplains or other religious ministers to offer that direction. Ironically, caregivers are eager to participate in formation programs. Invariably, their response is by exploring their own beliefs and understanding that they come to a deeper appreciation of their patients' concerns. Providing them with Biblical references provides the confidence that they can become proficient in "saying the right words." That is not to say they will now just quote scripture. The importance of this knowledge provides them insight into their own beliefs. This chapter aims to provide caregivers, family/support groups, and patients a foundation to reinforce their hope. For that reason, I provide a large amount of reference material to help understand scripture and the context in which it is written.

Aron Pinker poses the question, "Why does man have to die?" He answers the question by explaining that *the LORD God formed the man out of the dust of the ground and blew into his nostrils the breath of life, and the man became a living being* (Gn 2:7). It is not enough to form the human from the soil, but God must impart His divine breath into the person. After the "Fall," God, in His reckoning, returns humans to their original state: *You return to the ground – for from it you were taken. For dust you are, and to dust, you shall return* (Gn 3:19). Pinker postulates that we are put here for a purpose and then returned to our original state when our purpose on earth is fulfilled.[1] Pinker suggests that this description would subtly explain "dying" as God's taking back the "breath of life." What is from earth returns to earth, and what is from God

---

[1] Aron Pinker, "Job's Perspectives on Death," *Jewish Biblical Quarterly* 35, no. 2 (2007), 74.37.

returns to God.[2] This explanation makes the description of the "circle of life" reasonable. It is very similar to hearing a person explain that "when God is done with me on earth, then I am ready to return home." However, it does not tell us much about what happens after our purpose on earth is completed.

Throughout the ages, philosophers have had much to say about humanity's quest to bring meaning and purpose to their lives. Our view of human existence is influenced by Platonic, Neo-Platonic, and other Greek philosophical concepts. Christianity shares significant features with Platonism, the notion of self as divided between body and soul, with the soul more closely related to goodness and truth; this made Christianity's later soul-body division easier to understand. Both Christianity and Platonism assume absolute truth and unchanging reality; again, Plato's thought may have helped prepare Greek-speaking people for Christianity. Plato's heaven is one in which man is free from the imperfect physical, material world. The writings of Plato influenced such early church fathers as Clement of Alexandria. He saw Greek philosophy as the preparation for the Gentile understanding of the truth of Christ as the Mosaic Law prepared the Jewish people. Justin Martyr was also influenced by his study with Stoics, Aristotelians, Pythagoreans, and Platonists. He argued that God pre-

---

[2] Ibid.

pared the way for the revelation of Christ within Greek philosophy. Eusebius of Caesarea (263 CE) diligently sought to harmonize Plato with Christianity. Much like Plato, he believed that knowledge increases one's moral worth. Diarmaid McCullough quoted Eusebius, who says, "knowledge of God was found in the scripture and the writings of Aristotle and Plato: 'Philosophy is a preparation, making ready the way for him whom Christ is perfecting."[3] Finally, arguably the most influential early Church Father was Augustine, who was educated in Neo-Platonism, who in his work, *City of God*, proclaims that Platonists were near-Christians.[4] Plato's ideas concerning the nature of reality and the distinguishing of belief from opinion shaped Augustine's understanding of God as a source of absolute goodness and truth. Platonism helped Augustine to think of God as Spirit.

The discussion above is not so much designed to give a detailed description of Hellenist philosophy's influence on Christianity as it demonstrates the complex maturing progression of Christian thinking. In the book mentioned earlier, Coulter-Harris surveyed ancient Middle-Eastern, Egyptian, Greek, Indian, and Abrahamic religions to show how these earlier ways of thinking influenced how we view

---

[3] McCullough, 48.
[4] Ibid, 308.

immortality, the afterlife, and the human soul.[5] Like many before her, she determines that humans have always wondered what will happen to us at death. Most world religions share in a belief that the immortal soul lives on in some form. Like Voltaire, we can either conclude that "if God did not exist, it would be necessary to invent him" or take the approach that God created the world and its creatures purposely. Despite humanity's failings and weakness, God's plan, as revealed in the Bible and reflected upon in the Church's traditions and teachings, is one of a unifying creation that Dauphinais and Levering label, *Holy People, Holy Land*. God has a passion for restoring humankind to a state of original holiness. Dauphinais and Levering define holiness as a condition of balance and innocence before God and His creation. It provides a paradigm for God's intervention in human affairs, unifying sacred history as the record of God's reaching out to a world in need of grace. "Eternal life is the ultimate of holy people and holy land to which the entire Bible directs us."[6] With a Biblical view, I will now discuss how we try to make sense of human existence and the life hereafter.

---

[5] Coulter-Harris, 22.

[6] Michael Dauphinais and Matthew Levering, *Holy People, Holy Land: A Theological Introduction to the Bible* (Grand Rapids, MI: Brazos Press, 2005), 20.

We are not only curious about how we came to be but what will become of us finally. I intend to give examples from the Old and New Testaments and the thoughts of a few of the well-known Christian writers who have dared to address these profound questions about humanity's ultimate destiny. Dauphinais and Levering state that "the biblical story reveals that human beings were created to dwell harmoniously with God."[7] It is, namely, the story of how humanity seeks to identify meaning in life. For the believer, that effort culminates in Jesus' suffering and restoration of a right relationship with God in this life and the hereafter. Salvation History is the story of humans and the world they live in, seen as they seek purpose, meaning, and redemption from the time they come into existence until the *Day of the* LORD (1 Cor 15:23). The Parousia is when Christ, the world, and God will come together when God is *all in all* (1 Cor 15:28). The *Catholic Study Bible* notes state this verse means God's "reign is a dynamic exercise of creative power, an outpouring of life and energy through the universe, with no further resistance."[8] God can be fully God. Gerald O'Collins and Edward Farrugia

---

[7] Ibid, 10.

[8] Donald Senior, John J. Collins, and Mary Ann Getty-Sullivan, *The Catholic Study Bible: The New American Bible, Revised Edition*, Third (New York: Oxford University Press, 2016), 1621.

explain "that Salvation History is marked by ever-increasing expectations as divine promises point to future fulfillment."[9] The Second Vatican sees Salvation History as synonymous with the revelation history (*Dei Verbum* 2-4;14-15). For me, then, the discussion of "living as long as I can, as well as I can" begins with an effort to understand the divinely revealed message contained in Scripture.

The approach used in this examination of selected biblical literature will utilize scriptural interpretation tools that consider the various aspects of the passages through a theological perspective; that is one in which interpretation will, as Dauphinais and Levering term it, "flow from faith."[10] The historical-critical method provides a view of how we arrived at the text. It answers questions such as what is the original form, what does the text say, how did editors (redactors) affect the final form of the text, what is the particular genre used. Were written sources used, oral tradition included, how did the oral tradition finally come to be written, and what is the historical significance?

As described by the Pontifical Biblical Commission in a 1993 report to Pope John Paul II, the canonical approach extends the historical-critical analysis "by beginning from within an explicit framework of faith: The Bible as a

---

[9] Gerald O'Collins and Edward G. Farrugia, *A Concise Dictionary of Theology* (New York: Paulist Press, 2000), 234.

[10] Dauphinais and Levering, 20.

whole."[11] The report states, "The Bible is not a compilation of texts unrelated to each other; rather, it is a gathering together of a whole array of witnesses from one great tradition."[12] Typology, which is a way of interpreting events, people, and things in the Bible as foreshadowing a counterpart in the New Testament, will show the Old and New Testaments' connection and unity for salvation and the life hereafter. Isaiah's "Suffering Servant," for instance, is a clear example of foreshadowing the person of Jesus Christ's mission. I caution this is not an exhaustive survey; instead, it is a few examples to show how biblical writers spoke to the issue of human destiny. This method is best explained by referring to Pope Benedict XVI's *Verbum Domini,* in which he describes the necessities for understanding the divine aspect of the Bible. He writes:

Seeing that, in sacred Scripture, God speaks through human beings in human fashion, it follows that the interpreters of sacred Scripture, if they are to ascertain what God has wished to communicate to us, should carefully search out the meaning which the sacred writers had in mind, that meaning which God had thought

---

[11] Pontifical Biblical Commission, "The Interpretation of the Bible in the Church," *Origin,* April 23, 1993, http://www.catholic-resources.org/ChurchDocs/PBC_Interp.htm, 3.

[12] Ibid, 3.

well to manifest through the medium of their words."
On the one hand, the Council (Vatican II) emphasizes
the study of literary genres and historical context as
basic elements for understanding the meaning intended
by the sacred author. On the other hand, since Scripture
must be interpreted in the same spirit in which it was
written, the *Dogmatic Constitution* indicates three fundamental criteria for an appreciation of the divine dimension of the Bible:1) the text must be interpreted
with attention to the unity of the whole of Scripture;
nowadays this is called canonical exegesis; 2) account is
being taken of the living Tradition of the whole Church;
and, finally, 3) respect must be shown for the analogy of
faith. Only where both methodological levels, the historical-critical and the theological, are respected can
one speak of a theological exegesis, an exegesis worthy
of this book. (*VD* 34)

It is a method that requires close attention to the unity
of the Bible's message, how Old Testament passages can be
interpreted in light of the revelation of the New Testament,
and how such understanding has been applied to believers'
practices. Recognizing the Old and New Testament's unity
allows the reader to see people and events in the Old Testament as prefiguring the actions and words of Jesus Christ.
In biblical interpretation, it is a method to show how the
Old and New Testaments offer an understanding of God

and His connection to humans as one of love and mercy (forgiveness). It uses the tools of reason to come to a fuller understanding of faith. As St. Anselm of Canterbury wrote, it is an effort of "faith seeking understanding." For Anselm, as for us, understanding faith is only successfully accessed with the divine illumination derived from God's grace.

First, it must be noted that before the time of Jesus, it was problematic to comprehend that the God of the Jews could be so powerful and yet do such strange things as a walk in the Garden of Eden, argue with humans like Lot and Jonah and even wrestle with Jacob. How could God be both transcendent and immanent, powerful, and yet allow His people to suffer? Hellenized Jews of the diaspora (the scattering of Jews throughout the Greek-speaking world) began to interpret God's contradictory actions symbolically as the Greeks already gave to their writings. Thus, the Hellenized Jews were able to adapt the creation story to explain how God created the world out of nothing. 2 Maccabees 7:28 says, *I beg you, child, to look at the heavens and the earth and see all that is in them; then you will know that God did not make them out of existing things.* In the same way, humankind came into existence. God did not make them out of existing things: that is, all things were made solely by God's omnipotent will and creative word. This concept allowed the idea that God could remain divine (He created everything from nothing, *ex nihilo*) while entering into that same world He had created.[13]

Second, Coulter-Harris points to the idea of the soul, and the afterlife primarily came into the belief of Christianity from Greek and Egyptian mythology and philosophy.[14] The belief in the soul's immortality came to Jewish writers from contact with Greek philosophy, especially in Plato, as discussed earlier. Many writers contend that the Old Testament does not have a developed idea about the afterlife until the Babylonian Captivity and later writing in Daniel and Maccabees. The contention is that the writing about Sheol is a dark state or condition in which everyone exists at death. The opinion is that in the deuterocanonical period (Catholic term, Intertestamental for Protestants) after the prophets, Jewish thinking incorporated the Greek philosophical concepts of the immortality of the soul. My position is that the Old Testament foreshadows the more mature concept of the afterlife, culminating in humanity's final salvation through Christ's mediating grace. Thus, the examples I have chosen to use will reflect the idea that an understanding of what is meant by salvation results from taking earlier (Egyptian, Greek, Hebrew) concepts and in-

---

[13] Diarmaid MacCulloch, *Christianity: The First Three Thousand Years* (New York NY: Penguin Books, 2011), 69-70.

[14] Coulter-Harris, 1-2.

terpreting them in light of Christ's revealing presence within the world.

There are several examples of references to the afterlife in the Old Testament. John Bergsma and Brant Pitre provide several instances of allusion to life beyond earthly existence, including the prophecy of Baruch 2:27-35, Job 19:25-27, Ezekiel 37:1-14; Daniel 12:1-3; Ecclesiastes 11:7-12:7, and Wisdom 2-3.[15] Notation of the numerous references to an afterlife in the Psalms is then offered. A brief discussion of Isaiah's importance in the prefiguring of God's ultimate gift for human redemption will also be included.

Baruch links the prophecy of Moses that *the LORD, your God, will circumcise your hearts, and the hearts of your descendants* (Dt 30:6) with Jeremiah's assurance of a *new covenant* (Jer 31:31) to conclude that God has given His people an everlasting covenant (Bar 2:27-35). Baruch offers an explicit illustration of a belief that the dead have some form of an afterlife in the Prayer of the Dead: *LORD Almighty, God of Israel, hear the prayer of the dead of Israel, children who sinned against you; they did not listen to the voice of the LORD, their God, and their evils cling to us.* (Bar 3:4)

---

[15] John Sietze Bergsma and Brant James Pitre, A *Catholic Introduction to the Bible: The Old Testament,* (San Francisco: Ignatius Press, 2018), 632.

The idea that this verse reflects a belief in the afterlife may appear weak. Yet, it can be recalled that the souls of the dead are referred to as going down to Sheol. Sheol is described as devoid of love, hate, envy, work, thought, knowledge, and wisdom, which give purpose and meaning (Eccles 9:6; 9:10). Descriptions are dreary: there is no light (Job 10:21-22; 17:13; Ps 88:6; 88:12; 143:3), no memory (Ps 6:5; 88:12; Eccles 9:5), no praise of God (Ps 6:5; 30:9; 88:10-12; 115:17; Isa 38:18), in fact, no sound at all (Ps 94:17; 115:17). Its residents are entities without personality or strength, but worms, their eyes are dim, (Job 26:5; Ps 88:10-12; Isa 14:9-10) who can never hope to escape from its gates (Job 10:21; 17:13-16; Is 38:10). Sheol is like a predatory beast that swallows the living without being satisfied (Prov 1:12; 27:20; Isa 5:14). Some thought the dead were cut off from God (Ps 88:3-5; Is 38:11), while others believed that God's presence reached even to Sheol (Ps 139:8). These numerous mentions can be minimally seen as an allusion to an afterlife, even if it is a miserable destination. It appears to abrogate life with no meaning, purpose, joy, or interaction with others—non-being. Fortunately, God provides His people with an escape from this nonexistence.

Job 19:25-27 reads:

As for me, I know that my vindicator lives, and that he will at last stand forth upon the dust. This will happen when my skin has been stripped off, and from my flesh, I

will see God: I will see for myself, my own eyes, not an-
other's, will behold him: my inmost being is consumed
with longing. But you who say, "How shall we persecute
him, seeing that the root of the matter is found in him?

The word "vindicator" has also been translated from the
Hebrew word *goel* to mean "redeemer." The *Oxford Bible
Commentary* explains that this passage describes how Job is
looking for something or someone to call God to account
for His actions. This action suggests the entity is more po-
tent than a mediator or intercessor. The commentary pro-
poses three possible implications for Job's request. First, it
may be possible that a heavenly figure will champion Job's
cause after his death. Second, a divine character will allow
him (Job) to arise from the dead; or third, somehow Job
will be able to experience his vindication as some type of
ethereal entity.[16] What Job desires is to see God and survive
his encounter with evil. MacKenzie and Murphy argue the
implication is that Job will have a "survival of consciousness," which will connect Job to living with God after
death.[17] Although the Vulgate (Latin) translation presents

---

[16] James L Crenshaw, "Job," essay in *The Oxford Bible Commentary*, ed. John Barton and John Muddiman (Oxford, NY: Oxford University Press, 2007), pp. 342-343.

[17] R. A. MacKenzie, S.J. and Roland E. Murphy, O. Carm.,
"Job," essay in, *The New Jerome Biblical Commentary*, ed. Ray-

the idea of actual resurrection, which commentators now believe was not a line of thought that had matured at this time, nevertheless, there is a clear presentation that some form of life or consciousness survives after mortal life ends.

The *"Vision of the Dry Bones"* (Ez 37:1-14) is a symbolic description of God's creation of a new Israel. This vision summarizes Ezekiel's mission to the people exiled during the Babylonian king Nebuchadnezzar's deportation of royalty and leading citizens of Jerusalem. These exiles were overwhelmed with a sense of loss and sorrow. They were relocated to Tel-Abib (Ez 3:15), which was a destroyed city. The people who were deported were accustomed to a lifestyle of some comfort. Living among the ruins provoked bitterness and confusion. Gradually, they acclimate with many deportees gaining a level of well-being. They adopted Aramaic as the language and took Babylonian names for the months of the year. They did maintain their religion and national identity; they increasingly adapted to the dominant culture yet did not wholly abandon their traditions. Without the Temple in Jerusalem to offer sacrifice (the Temple was the only place for lawful sacrifice), the Law became the defining instrument for the faithful Jew. Theologically, the Law became central because of the people's stubborn breaking of the Law that brought on Jerusalem

---

mond E. Brown, Joseph A Fitzmyer, and Roland E. Murphy (Oxford University Press, 2007), 478.

and the Temple's destruction. To be restored, the Law must be upheld. Fidelity to the Law provided the people with the hope that a life of security and blessing would come to them if they were faithfully obedient. Faithfulness to the Law was a way to restore the relationship with God. It also opened the way for the idea that we are not burdened with the "guilt of his father": *If the son has done what is just and right and has been careful to observe all of my statues-he shall surely live!* (Ez 18:19). This passage indicates that we can be redeemed, through God's mercy, from the ultimate consequence of sin by acting in just and obedient ways.

In Ezekiel 37:1-14, there is a symbolic account of God's creation of a new Israel.

> *The hand of the* LORD *came upon me, and he led me out in the Spirit of the* LORD *and set me in the center of the broad valley. It was filled with bones. He made me walk among them in every direction. So many lay on the surface of the valley! How dry they were! He asked me: Son of man, can these bones come back to life?* "LORD GOD," *I answered,* "you alone know that." *Then he said to me: Prophesy over these bones, and say to them: Dry bones, hear the word of the* LORD! *Thus, says the* LORD GOD *to these bones: Listen! I will make breath enter you so you may come to life. I will put sinews on you, make flesh grow over you, cover you with skin, and put breath into you so you may come to life. Then you shall know that I*

am the LORD. I prophesied as I had been commanded. A sound started up, as I was prophesying, rattling like thunder. The bones came together, bone joining to bone. As I watched, sinews appeared on them, flesh grew over them, skin covered them on top, but there was no breath in them. Then he said to me: Prophecy to the breath, prophesy, Son of man! Say to the breath: Thus, says the LORD GOD: From the four winds come, O breath, and breathe into these slain that they may come to life. I prophesied as he commanded me, and the breath entered them; They came to life and stood on their feet, a vast army. He said to me: Son of man, these bones are the whole house of Israel! They are saying, "Our bones are dried up, our hope is lost, and we are cut off." Therefore, prophesy and say to them: Thus, says the LORD GOD: Look! I am going to open your graves; I will make you come up out of your graves, my people, and bring you back to the land of Israel. You shall know that I am the LORD, when I open your graves and make you come up out of them, my people! I will put my spirit in you that you may come to life, and I will settle you in your land. Then you shall know that I am the LORD I have spoken; I will do it—oracle of the LORD.

In the context in which the passage is presented, it is not foreshadowing resurrection. It promises to create a new ideal for the people in a hopeless situation shaped by the people's faithfulness to the covenant, which they were formerly unable to attain. Nevertheless, retrospectively, it is often referred to as foreshadowing the Christian doctrine of the resurrection and the afterlife. In Christian lectionaries, the passage is paired with Lazarus's rising in John 11:1-45 as an example of God's raising the dead. This combination makes a connection between God's power to bring a new life to an entire people, as the vision describes. That God, through Jesus' resurrection, offers a new life to believers is a connection that one can make with this story.

In again studying Job, we have the commentary of the suffering of a good man caused by the malicious actions of evil spirits permitted by God. We cannot know if we have true faith unless we are afflicted by suffering. Although it may appear to be an unsatisfactory description of why Job, or any faithful believer, must suffer, it also requires trust in God's divine will. It raises the question that if the present life requires some misery, does it mean we benefit from the afterlife? Job does not know why he is suffering; thus, the experience's redemptive worth is lost. He finds himself estranged from God. Job seems to see death as an escape from torment as he says in Job 14:13, *Oh, that you would hide me in Sheol, shelter me till your wrath has passed, fix a time to remember me.* Pinker says,

Job yearns to be in Sheol because "There the wicked cease from troubling and there the weary are at rest. All the prisoners are at ease; they hear not the voice of a taskmaster. Low and high is there, and slave is free of his master" (3:17-19). In Sheol, all are equal and finally at peace.[18]

Job's wish is for him to be like the tree (Jb 14:7-9) that can be renewed. Although Job 14:19 seems to destroy this hope, one can imagine that Job's "if only" lament is something that he believes God can make happen. One can see a hint of Job's belief that something can be experienced after death when Job first complains about his situation. There is a tranquility that he anticipates had he died at birth (Jb 3:11-13). He says, *For then I should have lain down and been at peace, with kings and counselors of the earth* (Jb 3:14-15a), suggesting some form of existence continues. For Job, death is seen as a place where he can escape from anguish and experience a level of calm and relief from suffering. In Sheol, wickedness ends; all are equal, yet there are no rewards for faithfulness or acting in a just manner. Although it is a solemn and even gloomy existence for Job, it beats the suffering he has endured in his mortal life. Moreover, it is a place of refuge where he can wait for God's rage

---

[18] Pinker, 75.

to diminish. This hopeful sentiment is alluded to in Job 14:13-17:

> *Oh, that you would hide me in Sheol, shelter me till your wrath is past, fix a time to remember me! If a man were to die and live again, all the days of my drudgery, I would wait for my relief to come. You would call, and I would answer you; you would long for the work of your hands. Surely then you would count my steps, and not keep watch for sin in me. My misdeeds would be sealed up in a pouch, and you would cover over my guilt.*

Job's reflection is merely wishful thinking if we look to Job 7:9-10, which says: *As a cloud dissolves and vanishes, so whoever goes down to Sheol shall not come up. They shall not return home again; their place shall know them no more.* This sentiment is repeated several times, including just before Job expresses his hopeful view in Job 14:13-17. Job wrestles with the idea of God and humans being in an interdependent relationship and yet one in which God has made life so intolerable that he seeks the relief of Sheol. How can God be just and merciful and, yet, not see Job's innocence? Yet Job can exclaim confidently during his time of misery and his longing for justice in Job 19:25-27:

> *That with an iron chisel and with lead, they were cut in the rock forever! As for me, I know that my vindicator*

lives and that he will at last stand forth upon the dust. This will happen when my skin has been stripped off, and from my flesh, I will see God: I will see for myself, my own eyes, not another's, will behold him: my inmost being is consumed with longing.

Job's story demonstrates a primitive idea of an afterlife, while not fully supporting resurrection. Nevertheless, it does establish that there was a concept that recognized an existence beyond mortal life.

The Book of Daniel promises delivery for the Jews out of their captor's hands (at this time carried out by Antiochus IV Epiphanes, a Hellenistic Greek king of the Seleucid Empire, 175 BCE -164 BCE). Some commentators contend that the book sets a timeline for the final resurrection. Nevertheless, it is the only book in the Old Testament that undoubtedly supports the awareness of personal resurrection: *Many of those who sleep in the dust of the earth shall awake; Some to everlasting life, others to reproach and everlasting disgrace* (Dn 12:2).

The *New American Bible* notes point out that Daniel's vision is not the universal resurrection developed later.[19] Daniel has a more limited view, which identifies two groups: the righteous who have suffered undeservedly will rise to eternal life. The wicked who have sinned without

_____

[19] Senior, RG 381.

punishment will be sentenced to "everlasting disgrace." In this passage, only these two groups are identified; all others will remain among the dead. In (12:3), Daniel identifies a select group of the righteous, *those with insight.* These are the wise ones who will lead others to lives of justice. For the righteous, physical death held the promise of resurrection to eternal life; for the unpunished sinner, physical death portends eternal retribution. As discussed in Ezekiel 37 and Isaiah earlier, prophecy uses language that suggests resurrection in talking about Israel's national restoration. Still, Daniel explicitly affirms the thought of personal resurrection.

Ecclesiastes accounts for humanity's effort to finding meaning and fulfillment in life. Qoheleth, the author of the Book of Ecclesiastes, tries to show how human reason cannot reconcile a pessimistic view in a world in which faith and obedience are essential to the well-being of the "chosen people." MacKenzie comments on that by observing that history shows that human events are cyclical with no real progress.[20] He sees temporal choices as not providing lasting happiness; injustice still prevails with the king's ruthless exploitation by taking their ancestral lands through unfair practices. Remember, the land was one of the promises made to Abraham by God and is now being revoked by the ruling elite. Qoheleth finally concludes that life cannot be

---

[20] MacKenzie, 478.

understood solely by reason. Humanity must come to have a right relationship with God for there to be purpose and meaning in life.

Ecclesiastes 1:14-18 gives a rather pessimistic view of life:

> *I have seen all things that are done under the sun, and behold, all is vanity and a chase after wind. What is crooked cannot be made straight, and you cannot count what is not there. Though I said to myself, "See, I have greatly increased my wisdom beyond all who were before me in Jerusalem, and my mind has broad experience of wisdom and knowledge," yet when I applied my mind to know wisdom and knowledge, madness, and folly, I learned that this also is a chase after wind. For in much wisdom, there is much sorrow; whoever increases knowledge increases grief.*

Although there is despair that death renders any success we attain in life meaningless, there is some flicker of hope for the righteous at the end of the book. Ecclesiastes 11:7-12:7 seems to balance the first section of the book by telling us that life is sweet, and one should enjoy it while we are able. He describes death in a way that echoes Genesis 2:7: *Out of the dust of the ground and blew into his nostrils the breath of life, and the man became a living being.* This inclusion lets us know that although our mortal bodies return to the dust from which they came, our breath returns to God for the righteous.

The Psalms is a collection of 150 sacred songs and poems that can be broadly classified into two genres: those that express lament and those that express positive balances to the lament by offering thanksgiving. The thanksgiving Psalms praise God in general for the creator's role or for a singular act of benevolence. The Psalms take the form of poems or hymns that are the expression of people's feelings. Provided below is a chart that shows some Psalm verses that deal with this eternal life and the genre in which they fit. A lament is a petitioner's request to have redress for a perceived injustice.

Psalm	Passage content	Genre
16:10	*For you will not abandon my soul to Sheol, nor let your devout one sees the pit.*	A lament that is a cry to God for deliverance.
30:2-4	*I praise you, LORD, for you raised me up, and did not let my enemies rejoice over me. O LORD, my God, I cried out to you for help, and you healed me. LORD, you brought my soul up from Sheol; you let me live, from going down to the pit.*	Thanksgiving for delivery from anguish.
30:12	*You changed my mourning*	Thanksgiving

	into dancing; you took off my sackcloth and clothed me with gladness. So that my glory may praise you and not be silent. O LORD, my God, forever will I give you thanks.	for God has delivered the psalmist from one state to the other.
37:37-40	*Observe the person of integrity and mark the upright; Because there is a future for a man of peace. Sinners will be destroyed together; the future of the wicked will be cut off. The salvation of the righteous is from the LORD, their refuge in a time of distress. The LORD helps and rescues them, rescues and saves them from the wicked because they take refuge in him.*	Thanksgiving prayer showing the consequences of the sinners' action while he provides refuge to the "person of integrity.
49:14-16	*This is the way of those who trust in themselves and the end of those who take pleasure in their own mouth. Like a herd of sheep, they will be put into Sheol, and death will shepherd them. Straight to the grave they descend, where their form will waste away,*	Thanksgiving for being rescued from Sheol and having one's life redeemed by God.

	Sheol will be their palace. But God will redeem my life, will take me from the hand of Sheol.	
61:2-5	*Hear my cry, O God, listen to my prayer! From the ends of the earth, I call; my heart grows faint. Raise me up, set me on a rock, for you are my refuge, a tower of strength against the foe. Let me dwell in your tent forever, take refuge in the shelter of your wings.*	This prayer is an expression of thanksgiving for God's providing protection in answer to prayer.
86:11-13	*Teach me, LORD, your way that I may walk in your truth, single-hearted, and revering your name. I will praise you with all my heart, glorify your name forever, LORD my God. Your mercy to me is great; you have rescued me from the depths of Sheol.*	Thanksgiving in the form of praise and gratitude for God's mercy
139:8	*If I ascend to the heavens, you are there; if I lie down in Sheol, there you are.*	Thanksgiving in the form of a meditation on God's omnipresence and omniscience, which offers protection.

I am confident that you could do an internet search and find many more examples that would support the awareness the writers of the Psalms had of God's intercession on behalf of those obedient to the Law and faithful to the "one God." Nevertheless, the examples given above demonstrate a rich tradition of belief in God's ability to save his people from everlasting damnation. The illustrations suggest after-life with God will come to the obedient and faithful.

The Old Testament foreshadowed the Christ savior figure, which brought us the promise of everlasting life through the Incarnate Word's sacrifice for humanity's freedom. Christ has been called the "last Adam," so Adam may be seen as prefiguring Christ. Abraham was asked to sacrifice his *only begotten son* (Gn 22:2), a term also used about Jesus (Jn 3:16). Only these two people are called an "only begotten son"—Christ and Isaac. The story of Abraham's sacrifice of his son Isaac demonstrates the great sacrifice being made by offering the Son as a gift to the world. Moses functions for Israel in the three conventional Old Testament roles of leadership: prophet, priest, and king—all of which are completed in Jesus Christ. Both deliver God's people from subjugation, act as a mediator, and above all, illuminate and make the Law active.

Another example is Jacob's beloved son, Joseph, with whom we find many parallels with Jesus. The following comparison strongly supports the idea that Joseph repre-

sents a revelation of that which was to come. Both Jesus
and Joseph are called beloved by their Fathers (Gn 37:3;
Mt 3:17). Both are hated out of jealousy and misunderstanding. His brothers hate Joseph because of his father's
favoring him (Gn 37:4), and Jesus is feared by the chief
priests (Mk 15:10). Joseph and Jesus both had an understanding that they would come to positions of power, but
not in a way that would subjugate others (Gn 37:7-10; Mt
26:64). They were both victims of a conspiracy to be mur-
dered (Gn 37:18-20; Mt 26:47-50, 66; Mk 14:26–15:47; Lk
22:39–23:56, and Jn 18:1–19:42). They were each abandoned, Joseph by his brothers and Jesus, most notably Peter (Gn 37:21-27; Mt 26:33-35; Mk 14:66-72; Lk 22:33-34;
Jn 13:36-38). Each was resisting temptation. Joseph defied
the wife of Potiphar, the Pharaoh's chief steward (Gn 39:7-
13), and Jesus resisted the temptation of Satan (Mt 4:1-11;
Mk 1:12-13; Lk 4:1-13). A final parallel is that both were
able to achieve glory, with Joseph being set over all of the
land of Egypt (Gn 4:41) and being made able to save his
people and Jesus in his resurrection and ascension to his
Father (Lk 24:50-53; Jn 20:17; Acts 1:1-12). These parallels
(and others not noted) illustrate how the Old Testament
foreshadowed Jesus' fulfillment of the final covenant with
God. Similar parallel comparisons could be made with Elisha and Elijah.[21]

---

[21] William Horbury, "The Wisdom of Solomon," essay, in,

The prophets Elijah and Elisha are credited with actions that are repeated and enlarged by Jesus. Elisha fed 100 men with only 20 loaves and some grain, with food left over much like Christ (2 Kgs 4:42–44); Elisha healed the sick (2 Kgs 5). Elijah and Elisha raised young boys from the dead (1 Kgs 17:21–22; 2 Kgs 4:32–35). Jesus feeds the multitude with bread and fish (5000 in Mt 14:13-21; Mk 6:31-44; Lk 9:12-17; Jn 6:1-14) (4000 in Mt 15:32-39; Mk 8:1-9) but more importantly with the words of eternal life. In John 6:3, Jesus tells us, *I am the bread of life. He who comes to me shall never hunger, and he who believes in Me shall never thirst.*

In the Old Testament, God is revealed, establishing a covenant. He did with Adam in the Garden, with Israel's nation through Moses, where the Law was delivered, with Noah after the great flood, Abraham and his descendants, and finally with King David. Restoration of a right relationship with God and eternal salvation are foundational in all the covenants. Each of these covenants was important and significant, and each one was fulfilled in the person of Jesus Christ. It is Christ who enables all humanity to come into reconciliation with God. Christ makes Abraham's family the chosen people who are the righteous seed to serve as the *light to the nations* (Is 49:6). Christ

---

The Oxford Bible Commentary, ed. John Barton and John Muddiman (Oxford, NY: Oxford University Press, 2007), 650.

confirms this fulfillment of the promise to Abraham in John 8:12 when he says, "I am the light of the world. Whoever follows me will not walk in darkness but will have the light of life." Christ makes the people of God the chosen people Moses commanded them to be by offering himself as the sacrifice for sin. Christ protects believers from all their enemies as *a sprout from the stump of Jesse* (Is 11:1). This image is a prophecy of God's deliverance in which Isaiah is certain to be speaking of the liberation of the Jewish people from exile. It is expanded further on in Chapter 11, where Isaiah predicts, "The root of Jesse, set as a sign for all the peoples--him the nations will seek out; his dwelling shall be glorious" (Is 11:10).

As can be noted from the preceding discussion, Isaiah's prophecy is an important connecting point between the Old and New Testaments concerning realizing the covenant between God and those faithful and obedient. For Christians, Isaiah's "Servant Songs" (Is 42:1-9; 49:1-7; 50:4-11; 52:13-53:12) is the prophecy of the coming of the LORD in the form of the Incarnate Word and eschatologically (at the end of time) that completes the restoration of Israel and extends redemption to all nations. Eschatological refers to the final events in the world's history and the ultimate destiny of the soul.[22] By Incarnate Word, I mean Jesus Christ, Son of God, who took on a physical, bodily

---

[22] Bergsma and Pitre, 158.

form. *And the Word became flesh and made dwelling among us* (Jn 1:14a). Although he was born of the mortal Mary, Jesus' earthly mother, he did not stop being divine. Although Jesus became fully human (Heb 2:17), he retained his status as God.

Isaiah gives us so much understanding of the Messiah's nature that it has often been called the "Fifth Gospel." Michael Canaris summarizes this idea when he writes:

> Since very early in Christianity's history, Isaiah's book has been a central text of our faith, even called by many patristic authors, the "Fifth Gospel." St. Jerome (c.342-420) claimed Isaiah "should be called an evangelist rather than a prophet because he describes all the mysteries of Christ and the church so clearly that you would think he is composing a history of what has already happened rather than prophesying about what is to come." Isaian concepts and terms that have become integral to Christian worship, texts, and iconography include, but obviously are not limited to: "beating their swords into plowshares and spears into pruning hooks" (2:4), "the wolf dwelling with the lamb" (11:6), "a voice crying out in the wilderness" (40:3), "a man of sorrows" (53:3), "a light to the nations" (42:6), "good news to the poor" (6:11), the "Prince of Peace" (9:6), a new heaven and a new earth" (65:17) and of course "the virgin shall

be with child, and bear a son, and shall name him Immanuel" (7:14).[23]

The early Christians used Isaiah in their evangelizing
work. Today the book of Isaiah is used extensively when the
word of God is proclaimed. The Catholic lectionary shows
322 verses of Isaiah are used in daily and Sunday Mass
readings. This number of verses is over 100 more than the
next most popular text from Sirach/Ecclesiasticus (208
verses used). The readings are prominent in Advent,
Christmas, Lent, Palm Sunday, Holy Thursday, Good Fri-
day, and Easter, as one would expect. Isaiah's prophesy is
vital in understanding God's promise of everlasting life and
how one can come to experience that gift.

Although there are allusions to the afterlife in the Old
Testament, as has been discussed, a refined notion of life
after death was given little interest before the Maccabees'
time. According to Diarmaid MacCulloch, the common
understanding that can be identified in the written texts
before the Babylonian exile is that human life comes to an
end for all but a few exceptional people.[24] The Maccabean

---

[23] Michael Canaris, "The Old Testament Book Known as the
Fifth Gospel," *Catholic Star Herald*, February 24, 2011,
https://catholicstarherald.org/the-old-testament-book-known-
as-the-fifth-gospel/.

[24] MacCulloch, 70.

War appears to have stimulated the development of belief in the afterlife, at least for those who had died so heroically. While this idea may not have been an entirely new concept, the Hellenized Jews now had Greek philosophy, particularly that of Plato, who talks of a human soul that could exist beyond mortal life.

The Old Testament story in 2 Maccabees 12:40-45 tells Judas Maccabeus's story of finding Jewish soldiers' corpses. They had been carrying *amulets sacred to the idols of Jamnia, which the law forbids the Jews to wear* (2 Mc 12:40). Thus, it was clear why these soldiers had fallen in battle on account of this sin. Judas nevertheless arranges for an offering of atonement to be made on their behalf. The author of 2 Maccabees says that Judas did so because:

"He then took up a collection among all his soldiers, amounting to two thousand silver drachmas, which he sent to Jerusalem to provide an expiatory sacrifice. In doing this, he acted in an excellent and noble way, since he had the resurrection in mind; for if he were not expecting the fallen to rise again, it would have been superfluous and foolish to pray for the dead. But if he did this with a view to the splendid reward that awaits those who had gone to rest in godliness, it was a holy and pious thought. Thus, he made atonement for the dead that they might be absolved from their sin." (12:43-46)

This story shows a clear resurrection concept and alludes to an intermediate state in which prayer is beneficial in atonement for the dead's sins.

Among the later Old Testament writers, Daniel 12:2-3 allows the idea of individual resurrection and life in an altered form.

> *Many of those who sleep in the dust of the earth shall awake; Some to everlasting life, others to reproach and everlasting disgrace. But those with insight shall shine brightly like the splendor of the firmament, and those who lead the many to justice shall be like the stars forever.*

The Book of Wisdom (Wisdom of Solomon), written near the time of Jesus, had a well-defined doctrine of immortality to confirm God's righteousness.[25] The book can be seen as an answer to the pessimism concerning an afterlife existence. Bergsma and Pitre express the idea that wisdom shows us that "righteousness finds its answer in the life to come."[26] The writer urges to seek wisdom through *righteousness or justice.* "It is only the righteous who will receive the gift of undying." (Wis 1:15). "It is the wicked who with hands and words invited death, consider it a

---

[25] Bergsma and Pitre, 668.
[26] Ibid, 670.

friend" (Wis 1:16). The wicked say we were born "by mere chance" (Wis 2:2), that human reason is merely a material and physiological process, that pleasure in the here and now is what counts, and that strength and power are the means for establishing right and wrong (Wis 2:11).

The Book of Wisdom also demonstrates the desire to persecute the righteous who obstruct the wicked world view. Wisdom 2:10 identifies this aspiration: "*Let us oppress the righteous poor; let us neither spare the widow nor revere the aged for hair grown white with time.*" The writer then gives us a description of the persecution and death of the blameless person that parallels the passion of Jesus.

Let us lie in wait for the righteous one, because he is annoying to us; he opposes our actions, reproaches us for transgressions of the Law, and charges us with violations of our training. He professes to have knowledge of God and styles himself a child of the LORD. To us, he is the censure of our thoughts; merely to see him is a hardship for us. Because his life is not like that of others, and different are his ways. He judges us debased; he holds aloof from our paths as from things impure. He calls blest the destiny of the righteous and boasts that God is his Father. Let us see whether his words be true; let us find out what will happen to him in the end. For if the righteous one is the Son of God, God will help him and deliver him the hand of his foes. With violence and torture, let us put

him to the test that we may have proof of his gentleness
and try His patience. Let us condemn him to a shameful
death; for according to his own words, God will take care
of him. (Wis 2:12-20)

Even with this persecution and murder of the righteous
person, the writer reveals that death is not their end. Using
the canonical criticism method, we can see how Ecclesiastes
and Wisdom's books help understand wisdom interpretation's maturation. Canonical Criticism is an analysis that
shows how biblical books interrelate. Our examination
shows how the Book of Wisdom answers life after death,
which was presented in Ecclesiastes. In Wisdom 3:1-12, we
are told that the righteous only seem to have died; actually,
God has found them worthy and has taken them to himself.
The author establishes that for the righteous suffering allows that *[i]n their time of judgment when they shall shine*
and dart about as sparks through stubble (Wis 3:7). Explicitly, they will experience God's loving judgment. For the
righteous, suffering will be a time of refinement and an opportunity to display their faithfulness to God's will. On the
other hand, for the evil person suffering is truly divine punishment from which there is no escape.

The author sees wisdom as the "primary divine agent
for salvation present and acting in the history of God's people from Creation through Exodus," which continues to-

day.[27] Wisdom is an essential requirement for just people. It is illustrative of those who represent a way of reasoning and behaving, which is orderly, communally sensitive, and morally principled. Thus, righteousness is the operationalizing of wisdom, which leads to immortality. Wisdom 6:17-20 shows the relationship between wisdom and everlasting life.

> *For the first step toward wisdom is an earnest desire for discipline; then, care for discipline is love of her; love means the keeping of her laws; To observe her laws is the basis for incorruptibility, and incorruptibility makes one close to God; thus, the desire for wisdom leads to a kingdom.*

Later, we see that the kingdom that is identified in Wisdom 6:20 is the kingdom of God (Wis 1:10), in which "She" (Wisdom) shows Jacob the Kingdom of God.[28] The writer is showing that the kingdom that wisdom leads us to is the kingdom of God.

The period in which the Book of Wisdom was written is after Alexander the Great (336-323 BCE) during his successors' reign, the Ptolemies (a Hellenistic kingdom ruled out of Egypt), and the Seleucids (a state carved from the Greeks'

---

[27] Ibid, 675.

[28] Ibid, 674.

empire). This timeframe, called the Hasmonean Period, was when the Maccabees defeated the Greeks (167 BCE) and ruled Judea in semi-autonomy from the Seleucids. This period lasted for approximately 100 years. The Hasmoneans, Egyptian, Greek, and Hebrew thinking influenced ideas concerning immortality and the afterlife. The author of the Book of Wisdom made use of the concept of the worth of divine wisdom. The description of wisdom is drawn from the Jewish traditions, from the cult of the Egyptian God Isis (goddess of wisdom), and Hellenistic philosophy. Bergsma and Pitre contend that the Book of Wisdom "provides us with what is easily the most detailed description of life after death in the Old Testament."[29]

The writer contrasts the righteous and their reward to that which comes to the wicked in Wisdom 1:15-16 when he writes: *For righteousness is undying. It was the wicked who, with hands and words, invited death, considered it a friend, and pined for it, and made a covenant with it because they deserve to be allied with it.* Undying—that is immortality—is not seen as a characteristic of the soul. Instead, it is a gift from God. The writer takes a Greek concept of an immortal soul and places it in a Jewish context of God's covenant relationship. The wicked of the world are those whose goal in life appears to maximize physical pleasure even at others' expense. Their actions result in materialistic (Wis

---

[29] Ibid, 679.

2:3), hedonistic (Wis 2:7), and relativistic (Wis 2:11) behavior.[30]

Wisdom then shows how the wicked seek to persecute the righteous, then describes how wisdom can overcome evil.

> *For she is a reflection of the eternal light, untarnished mirror of God's active power, and image of his goodness. Although she is alone, she can do everything; herself unchanging, she renews the world, and, generation after generation, passing into holy souls, she makes them into God's friends and prophets; for God loves only those who dwell with wisdom. She is indeed more splendid than the sun, she outshines all the constellations; compared with light, she takes first place, for light must yield to night, but against wisdom, evil cannot prevail.* (Wis 7:26-30)

Wisdom and righteousness are the ways that lead to immortality: *thus, the desire for wisdom leads to the kingdom* (Wis 6:20). The kingdom spoken of here is the "kingdom of God" for which wisdom shall rescue the righteous from persecution.

> *But wisdom rescued from tribulations those who served her. She, when a righteous man fled from his brother's*

---

[30] Ibid.

*anger, guided him in right ways, showed him the king-
dom of God, and gave him knowledge of holy things; She
prospered him in his labors and made abundant the fruit
of his works. Stood by him against the greed of his de-
frauders, and enriched him; She preserved him from foes
and secured him against ambush, and she gave him the
prize for his hard struggle that he might know that devo-
tion to God is mightier than all else. She did not abandon
a righteous man when he was sold, but rescued him from
sin. She went down with him into the dungeon, and did
not desert him in his bonds, until she brought him the
scepter of royalty and authority over his oppressors,
proved false those who had defamed him, and gave him
eternal glory.* (Wis 10: 9-14)

Not only did wisdom rescue the righteous, *but when an
unrighteous man withdrew for her in his anger, he perished
in his fratricidal wrath* (Wis 10:3). While this chapter of
Wisdom deals with the Israelites' relationship to God in
Genesis, it has clear parallels to Jesus' saving power for believers.

Summary

The chapter has offered a good deal of contextual background and scriptural references that point out how the
Judeo-Christian view of right living and preparation for full

communion with the Creator evolved. God's plan of salvation that is ultimately fulfilled in the Incarnation is revealed within the scriptures. A close reading of scripture utilizing the methods of interpretation that are the product of God's gift of intellect and reasoning to humans allows us to use the scripture to bring comfort, support, and hope to our neighbors. This is especially true for "those most in need of thy mercy" (from the Fatima Petition in the Rosary prayer).

The section has focused on the human belief in a life hereafter, which is present through history in different cultural myths and religious beliefs. One cannot empirically (through means of observation) know about life after death other than descriptions of resuscitations described in ancient writings (including the Bible). Nevertheless, philosophers and theologians throughout the ages, including the present time, have used reason to speculate (conjecture without firm evidence) that forces transcend nature, which we call God. Blaise Pascal used what is termed "Pascal's Wager" as a practical argument for belief in God. In his *Pensées*, Pascal used the following contention to show that belief in the Christian religion is rational: "If the Christian God does not exist, the agnostic loses little by believing in him and gains correspondingly little by not believing. If the Christian God does exist, the agnostic gains eternal life by believing in him and loses an infinite good by not believing."[31] Admittedly, Pascal used this argument to convert his friends who had rejected religion and lived immorally. This section is not designed to convert. Instead, it establishes that belief in a power beyond human capability and frailty is reasonable.

Moreover, the message of those who teach morality based upon such precepts as the Ten Commandments and the Sermon on the Mount (or Plain in Lk 6:20-49) will create a world in which we can begin to experience God's *kingdom on earth as it is in heaven* (Mt 6:10). By doing so, we prepare ourselves for that time when we experience what Thomas Aquinas termed the *"beatific vision,"* which is the human being's "final end" in which one reaches perfect happiness. "Wherefore God alone can satisfy the will of man, according to the words of Psalms 102:5: *Who satisfieth thy desire with good things.* God alone constitutes man's happiness" (ST I–II, 2, 8).[32] Such happiness cannot be found in material or physical pleasure alone. It can only exist in God's everlasting perfection.

---

[31] Ibid, 670-671.

[32] "Les Provinciales," *Encyclopædia Britannica* (Encyclopædia Britannica, inc.), accessed February 21, 2021, https://www.britannica.com/biography/Blaise-Pascal/Les-Provinciales#ref365135.

Selected Reading

A Catholic Introduction to the Bible: The Old Testament, by John Bergsma and Brant Pitre, is a good reference source to demonstrate how the Old and New Testaments form one continuous whole.

Holy People, Holy Land, A Theological Introduction to the Bible by Michael Dauphinais and Matthew Levering uses what they term a theological reading of the Scripture to describe how God intends to lead his people into a complete state of holiness.

In the Beginning: A Catholic Understanding of the Story of Creation and the Fall, by Pope Benedict XVI (Joseph Ratzinger) presents the creation story in a balanced understanding of biblical writings that avoid the pitfalls of literalists as well as rationalist interpretations of the story.

Chapter Four

Paul and Other Cultural Influences on Christianity

For to me, life is Christ,
death is gain. If I go on living in the flesh,
that means fruitful labor for me. (Philippians 1:21-22)

The previous chapter demonstrated that the concept of an afterlife and immortality results from a process of evolution and development of thought that incorporated the ideas from various Mediterranean cultures, notably including Egyptian, Greek, and Hebrew cultural and philosophical traditions. This chapter will explore the influence of the Mediterranean world in more detail. I will use a few examples to illustrate how the various cultures influenced how we interpret what is finally realized in Jesus Christ's person. These ideas helped to bring clarity to the true significance of Jesus Christ in the salvation of humanity. I then look at the teaching of Paul concerning our ultimate destiny. To fully understand God's message, one needs to show how what Christianity says about morality is inclusive of humanity's moral teachings. Besides, it is vital to understand what Paul taught is the most significant scriptural influence on Christianity. The chapter concludes with a brief discussion of the Gospel writers view of Jesus' role in salvation history.

There can be little doubt that Egyptian mythology concerning the afterlife can be shown to impact Judaism and later Christianity. Genesis tells Jacob's family's story, the sale of his beloved son Joseph into slavery, and the family's ultimate rescue from famine and reuniting with Joseph in Egypt. Joseph was elevated to Vizier's central position, the second most influential role in Egypt next to the Pharaoh because of his unmatched ability to interpret dreams. We later find the Israelites fall into disfavor and for 400 years are in slavery in Egypt. During this long residence in Egypt, it is inconceivable that they did not contact the Osiris story, which offered the hope of new life, initially only to royalty, to and later for all people. The Egyptian concept of the soul or spirit being disconnected from the body at death yet maintaining its personal qualities as it took up residence in the sky with God influences both Judaic and Christian faith.[1]

Also, there is a time of judgment in which rewards and punishment were meted out based upon their actions during their mortal lives, prefiguring the Christian view of God's final judgment. The mythology developed around the idea of the Pharaoh as a god. The belief that any insult to the Pharaoh was an affront to the gods strengthened the

---

[1] Coulter -Harris, 22.

role's power. Although ordinary people could not become gods, their souls could obtain immortality. Again, while not showing the Pharaoh as a mediator to the gods for the people, this concept did show that belief in his divinity was required to allow immortality.

The Egyptians had another concept called "second death," which carried the penalty of final and irrevocable death from which there can be no salvation. In the first death, the person experienced many of the same things they had in their temporal life as they awaited the final judgment. The idea of a second death held that only the most wicked, entirely valueless persons would suffer dying a second time. Notably, the Roman Catholic Church and some other Christian sects seem to use this concept to reinforce the view of a tortured existence for unbelievers in the afterlife. The first death was passing, sleeping until the resurrection of the body, and final judgment. The second death, in this model, is eternal damnation.[2]

The Hebrew view of the soul was a part of humans' temporal unity, composed of a body and a soul. Jewish concepts of the soul are subject to a combined view that ascribes no metaphysical significance to human existence; it sees in humans only their actual body and sees the soul simply as the element that gives the body its vitality. The soul is the site of emotions but not a spiritual life separate

---

[2] Ibid, 24.

from the body or mental or emotional life in conflict with the body. It is where feelings and desires, physical as well as spiritual, are located.

Ancient Greek writing and religion had gods being among humans, which is similar to God walking with Adam and Eve, reinforcing the notion that gods and immortal beings walked the earth. More importantly, the Greeks developed philosophies about the soul's existence that become integral parts of Christian theology. The early Church writers favored Platonism because of "its clear doctrine of transcendence, the idea that there is a single (divine) principle upon which all things depend."[3] Aristotle later teaches that the soul exists as the form of the body.

In the West, Aristotle was favored because "his analysis of the structure of finite beings (including humans) seemed to provide a good account of nature to complement revelation's account of grace."[4] Both of these philosophers opened the way to seeing knowledge as a way of allowing humans to understand our relationship to God better. While Plato remained the primary philosophical influence

---

[3] Aidan Nichols, *The Shape of Catholic Theology: An Introduction to Its Sources, Principles, and History* (Collegeville, MN: The Liturgical Press, 1991), 49.

[4] Peter Kreeft, *A Shorter Summa: The Most Essential Philosophical Passages of St. Thomas Aquinas' Summa Theologica* (San Francisco, CA: Ignatius Press, 1993), 149.

on the early Christian theologians, Aristotle's concepts were the most often used methodology in refining theological thought.[5] Aristotle's use of logic gave theologians the tools to analyze the Scripture of the Church Fathers' writing. It emerged from the use of logic in the form of syllogisms to interpret Scripture and early writings. Theology is expressed as problems or questions. The influence of Greek thinkers, particularly Plato and Aristotle, profoundly changed the way of looking at the soul from the Hebrew idea. It paved the way for interpreting the Incarnation's significance that allowed Christianity to become a widespread belief. Indeed, the Hebrew concept of a covenant relationship with God and these two philosophers greatly impacted Christianity as we see it unfold in the New Testament, especially in Paul's letters.

Paul and the Gospel writers of Christianity

A review of New Testament teaching will focus on Saul of Tarsus, who became known as Paul, due to his continuing impact on Christianity. Paul reports that he was a persecutor of the Christians as a Pharisaic Jew. There are several reports of his conversion experience in Acts. The first account in Acts 9:1-18 is told by Luke as a first-hand, actual account of the event. The second description in Acts 22:6-

---

[5] Ibid.

16 describes his testimony during his trial before the Jews. After years of preaching throughout Asia Minor and Greece, Paul had returned to Jerusalem. He was falsely accused of bringing Timothy, a Gentile, into the Temple, and he was arrested. Addressing his accusers, Paul reflected on his conversion, telling them that he was a Jew, raised in the diaspora but educated under the famous Jewish teacher Gamaliel. There is some question as to the accuracy of Luke's biography on this point. He recounted his zeal for persecuting Christians and his mission to Damascus. The third version of the story, Acts 26:12-20, differs from the other two. Paul had been in prison for over one year, and he had been testifying in his defense before the Judean king Agrippa. In this version, Paul is directed by Jesus to bring the gospel to the Gentiles. In Paul's letters, Jerome Murphy-O'Connor describes the description of his conversion as "dismayingly discreet."[6] In 1 Corinthians 9:1, Paul gives an emotionally charged defense of his right to be considered an apostle when he says, *Am I not free? Am I not an apostle? Have I not seen our LORD? Are you not my work in the LORD?* In 1 Corinthians 15, Paul, while offering his audience the teaching about Christ's resurrection appearances, provides the following proof statement: *Last of all, as to one born abnormally, he appeared to me* (1 Cor 15:8). In Galatians 1:11-16, Paul also speaks of the revelation of Jesus

---

[6] Ibid, 287.

Christ during his call, which he sees as a command to proclaim the mission of Jesus Christ to the Gentiles. Paul sees the revelation of Jesus Christ and an invitation to ministry as connected.

Paul is unique in that he is steeped in the law and understanding of God's covenant relationship as a Pharisaic Jew. The latter is aware of Greek philosophy and religious mythology through his education and status as a Roman citizen. Initially, Paul is seen in a leading position among those who saw the entry into eternal life is tied to the law's observance. The Law was understood to cover three areas: ceremonial law, relating to forms of worship (Leviticus); civil law, dictating daily living (Deuteronomy); and moral laws, which are direct commands of God. A good example is the Ten Commandments (Ex 20:1-17). Paul's revelation turns him from adherence to the Law and a structure of works of righteousness to a message centered "on the grace of God and justification by faith."[7] Paul is often portrayed as adopting the Greek way of thought as he brought the message of Jesus to the Gentiles. Yet, Meister and Stumpf argue that Paul's ideas about "justification and salvation, his eschatology and emphasis on the resurrection, and his

---

[7] Jerome Murphy-O'Connor, *Paul a Critical Life* (Oxford: Oxford University Press, 2012), 71.

instructions about spiritual life and practice" continue to reflect Paul's Jewish heritage.[8]

Paul's post-Damascus revelation concerning Jesus' resurrection is most important to review as part of the conversation about New Testament eschatology (concerned with the final events in humanity's history). Before Paul's revelatory experience, he was among those who saw the covenant being fulfilled when the Jewish people were freed from their oppressors. This emancipation would signify that they had been redeemed. For Paul, the time of vindication had not yet come because there was no Messiah. His clash with the Christians turned on his understanding of their teachings as heretical. Identifying Jesus as the Messiah was illogical since he was crucified, "hung on a tree," and therefore cursed. Paul's (known as Saul) motivation was to correct this false teaching within Judaism; for him, the Messiah would come to free all of Israel. He probably saw himself as a reformer, working within the existing religious system, to deal sharply with the followers of a person who had desecrated the Temple and died in the disgrace of crucifixion (the death of a common criminal) at the hands of the Romans. His concern was for the Jewish community's well-being: the worship of Jesus threatened Roman authority.[9]

---

[8] Chad V. Meister and J. B. Stump, *Christian Thought: A Historical Introduction* (London: Routledge, 2017), 53-54.

[9] Ibid, 54.

When Paul encounters the resurrected Jesus, he sees that God's action with Jesus signifies that the teaching concerning Jewish eschatology was faulty. The notion of one person experiencing the resurrection alone before the end of history was unthinkable before the Apostles and their followers began proclaiming that it was what had already happened. Paul's encounter with the risen Christ was a clear sign that the last days had arrived. Moreover, Jesus had instructed Paul to take the good news to the Gentiles. He identifies this as the mission for which Christ has called him.

Now I want you to know, brothers, that the gospel preached by me is not of human origin. For I did not receive it from a human being, nor was I taught it, but it came through a revelation of Jesus Christ. For you heard of my former way of life in Judaism, how I persecuted the Church of God beyond measure and tried to destroy it, and progressed in Judaism beyond many of my contemporaries among my race, since I was even more a zealot for my ancestral traditions. But when [God], who from my mother's womb had set me apart and called me through his grace, was pleased to reveal his Son to me so that I might proclaim him to the Gentiles, I did not immediately consult flesh and blood. (Gal 1:11-16)

This passage is a clear allusion to Paul seeing himself called a prophet in the manner of Jeremiah, who was also called while still in his mother's womb (Jer 1:5). In Galatians 3:28-29, Paul declares all *are one in Christ Jesus. And, if you belong to Christ, then you are Abraham's offspring, heirs according to the promise.* Paul teaches that those who become one with Jesus Christ will share his resurrection and everlasting life in glory.

This teaching then begs the question, how does one achieve being one with Jesus Christ. In other words, how can one be saved? Paul saw salvation coming through a proper relationship with God, which is being justified. Paul does not see a forensic justification where God passes judgment as we so often view the term today. Significantly, Paul believed that through the power of the message of Christ's death on the cross and resurrection that the community would become Christians through initiation in baptism and sharing of a common way of life. Paul's message was not a method concerning how to become a Christian. It was a message in which he shared the good news revealed to him that through the cross and resurrection, Jesus was LORD. Salvation was a gratuitous gift from God, one made from grace available to all who came to believe. Often lost in the idea that we are saved by the grace of God, with faith being the only requirement, is Paul's stress on *whoever is in Christ is a new creation: the old things have passed away; behold, new things have come* (2 Cor 5:17). There is a new covenant; it is a call to a different way of life in which Christians *no longer live for themselves, but for him who died for their sake died and was raised* (2 Cor 5:15).

Paul uses athletic metaphors to show how Christians establish and maintain habits such as fasting, prayer, and abstinence as ways to become more righteous. Righteousness is something that comes through faith but can be reinforced by good habits. Paul is clear in Romans 3:21-31 that it is not works of the Law that justify, but by God's grace that we are redeemed. By this, Paul is referring to ritual, ceremonial, and religious observance laws of the Jews. Paul's vision is one of Christians becoming a community that is part of the kingdom of God both here and now and as will be in heaven.

Paul should also be viewed from the perspective that he believed the end of time was near at hand, and he had a clear vision for how we will appear in the life hereafter. 1 Corinthians 15:20-27 describes Paul's image of the order in which the end will come when he writes:

Brothers and sisters: Christ has been raised from the dead, the first fruits of those who have fallen asleep. For since death came through man, the resurrection of the dead came also through man. For just as in Adam all die, so too in Christ shall all be brought to life, but each one in proper order: Christ the firstfruits; then, at his coming, those who belong to Christ; then comes the end, when he hands over the kingdom to his God and Father, when he has destroyed every sovereignty and every authority and power. For he must reign until he has put all his enemies under his feet. The last enemy to be destroyed is death, for "he subjected everything under his feet.

There have been arguments made that Paul's notion of imminence was not that clearly defined. Some claim he believed the end would come within the lifetime of the readers. Others point to the lack of specificity using 1 Thessalonians 5:2, where Paul says, *You yourselves know very well that the day of the* LORD *will come like a thief in the night.* Later in the same pericope, he urges the followers to be vigilant and stay alert and sober. In Romans 13:11-12, Paul tells his audience:

And do this because you know the time; it is the hour now for you to awake from sleep. For our salvation is nearer now than when we first believed; the night is advanced, the day is at hand. Let us then throw off the works of darkness [and] put on the armor of light.

These two verses are set within Romans in Chapters 12-15, an everyday appeal that presumes the Torah is no longer the sole standard of conduct. Paul lays out a "blueprint" for promoting a life of peace and harmony among all believers. This model for living is important to Paul because, for him, the final days have begun. The specific laws of Judaism have been modified and even done away with in the service of converting the Gentiles. Paul sees the *ekklesiai* (community of believers) as those whom their faith has saved. Paul believed Christian principles were necessary because the time of the second coming was near.

The idea of the "time is near" is also expressed in 1 Corinthians 7:29-31 when he writes:

I tell you, brothers, the time is running out. From now on, let those having wives act as not having them, those weeping as not weeping, those rejoicing as not rejoicing, those buying as not owning, those using the world as not using it fully. For the world in its present form is passing away.

In this passage, Paul advises approaching ordinary life activities that do not focus on the material or transitory elements of life. His message is to turn to God. Jesus will rescue us from the fury expected for those who have not embraced the new age. In 1 Thessalonians, Paul addresses the group's concern that some of their members had already died. He reassures them that those who have *fallen asleep* (1 Thes 4:13–18) will be raised again at the coming of the LORD. It appears Paul eagerly looks to the second coming with high expectations. He anticipates it happening within his lifetime; he does not predict a specific time. Instead, he urges believers to be ready—that they have a sense of urgency.

While some scholars suggest that Paul's view of the imminence of the end times was faulty, it is hard to argue with his teaching regarding preparation for that time. Paul's reading of the signs of the end times, which came from the revelatory experience of seeing the risen Christ along with the call to convert the Gentiles, was the indicator for his prescient proclamation. It was his personal experience of Christ's resurrected body that propelled his ministry.

It is important to note that Paul gives us a vivid description of seeing Jesus. Garry Wills states in his book, *What Paul Meant*, that "of all those who saw the risen LORD, Paul is the only one whose words we possess."[10] The other descriptions we read have Jesus in variable situations, such as eating food with others and materializing and dematerializing. For instance, Jesus is often not recognized, as with Mary Magdalene at the tomb (Jn 20:14-15). She mistook him for the gardener until he spoke, or on the road to Emmaus, the two travelers do not recognize Jesus until he had a meal with them, and then Jesus again disappears (Lk 24:31). After the fact, these stories are told by a secondary (one that interprets or analyzes events originally occurring

---

[10] Karen Armstrong, *St. Paul: The Apostle We Love to Hate* (Boston: New Harvest, Houghton Mifflin Harcourt, 2015), 23.

elsewhere) source. Paul is the only one who tells us how the risen LORD appears.

In 1 Corinthians 15:8, Paul states that Jesus *appeared to me.* Unlike Luke's account of Paul's encounter, he sees nothing but a flash of light (Acts 9:3-8, 22:6-11, 26:13-19). Wills describes it as a *photism* (burst of light) followed by an audition (a disembodied voice), which is different from the Gospel stories that consist of supernatural experiences of a physical presence in which participants interact with the apparition.[11] Paul's account is then consistent with the other apostles' experiences and those close to Jesus who interacted with Jesus post-resurrection. Moreover, Paul gives us a description of how the risen body appears through the use of analogies. In 1 Corinthians 15:35-55, he uses the analogy of a seed in which one form must change for the plant to emerge. Paul teaches that the body becomes qualitatively different after death. We are animated by natural forces that include corruptibility, weakness, and spiritual frailty during our temporal life. After our death and subsequent resurrection, we assume qualities that are properties of God, including incorruptibility and spiritual strength. In other words, we are sown as a natural body and raised as a spiritual body (1 Cor 15:44).

---

[11] Garry Wills, *What Paul Meant* (New York: Viking, 2006), 21.

Paul then uses the analogy of the first Adam who came from the earth; the second Adam, Jesus, came from heaven. Just as we bear the image of the first Adam, we can be transformed into the image of the Son. Paul associates his encounter with Jesus as the model in which he will change our lowly body to conform with his glorified body by the power that enables him *to bring all things into subjection to himself* (Phil 3:21). Paul speaks knowingly about how he understands life hereafter because he has seen the splendor of Jesus' face.

Because he has had a real experience with the risen Lord, Paul realizes that Jesus is the center of salvation history. In 1 Corinthians 15:12-14, he writes:

Now, if Christ is proclaimed as raised from the dead, how can some of you be saying that there is no resurrection of the dead? If there is no resurrection of the dead, then Christ cannot have been raised either, and if Christ has not been raised, then our preaching is without substance, and so is your faith.

In this statement, Paul shows that he is "all in" because he has evidence from his encounter with the risen Lord. Paul's story is essential in this book because his faith is based on the certainty of Jesus' being the fulfillment of God's promise not just to the Jewish people but to the entire world. His commitment is based on first-hand knowledge of the risen LORD and the messages he received, which pointed him to reach out to the Gentiles, despite the difficulties this would ultimately present to him.

Paul, unlike the Gospel writers, does not focus on Jesus' works or even his teaching. His ministry is the sure sign he has experienced Jesus' resurrection. Paul preaches the end times inaugurated by Jesus' presence and glorification, then realized and anticipated in believers' experience through the Spirit (Rom 8:11-13; 1 Cor 6:14; 2 Cor 1:21-22, 5:5). Paul teaches that God is preparing us for the resurrected bodily life through the Spirit's gift, which comes through baptism. Paul provides us with a faith model that includes suffering and is filled with great joy and anticipation of the day of splendor when we are all raised and brought to God's side.[12] While Paul is a pivotal figure in understanding the Christian view of eternal life, some mention needs to be made concerning how the other Gospel writers understood the LORD's coming.

For the Gospel writers, Jesus was proof that the kingdom of God had been inaugurated through the actions of his healing, casting out of demons, ability to forgive sin, and teaching of love and reconciliation. The coming kingdom would be when God's will *be done on earth as it is in heaven* (Mt 6:10). The Gospel writers showed Jesus' teaching and preaching as one of good news with the extension

---

[12] Ibid, 20.

of the Jewish concept of judgment on those who are evil. Evildoers were those that corrupted the Temple and rejected Jesus' message of love. Evil is defined in terms of the response to Jesus or his teachings. The day of judgment is set as being when the faithful and unfaithful will be separated. David Wenham concludes that Jesus anticipated his departure as demonstrated in the prediction passages (Mt 16:21-23, 17:22-23, 20:17-19; Mk 8:31-32, 9:30-32, 10:32; Lk 9:43-45, 18:31-34; Jn 8:27-30, 12:7-8, 12:23, 14:26-31) and anticipated that the disciples would continue his work here on earth until He returned to complete the kingdom of God.[13]

Clear evidence of the concept that Jesus inaugurated the end times and ultimate power over the dead's fate in John 5:19-30. In that pericope, Jesus claims authority given to him by God to give life to whomever he wishes and gives all judgment to the Son, so the Son may be honored as is the Father (Jn 5:22-23), which is a clear indication of his inaugurated signal of the end time. In verses 5:27-30, John shows that Jesus has authority over not just the living but also the dead. In these passages, John has demonstrated Jesus' having power over life and death now as well as the future. If Paul and the Gospel writers saw Jesus as the beginning of the end, they likely saw the end as imminent.

----

[13] David Wenham, *Paul: Follower of Jesus or Founder of Christianity?* (Grand Rapids: Eerdmans, 1996), 294.

John the Baptist, according to Matthew 3:2, exhorts his followers to *repent, for the kingdom of heaven is at hand.* Matthew and Luke use the same metaphor of the ax lying at the tree's root with those not producing good fruit thrown into the fire (Mt 3:30; Lk 3:9). These are warnings of a looming time of judgment. Wenham points out that:

> More specifically, the Gospels have several sayings of Jesus in which he speaks specifically of things happening soon, notably Mt 10:23: "You will not have gone through all the towns of Israel before the Son of Man comes, "Mt.16:28; Mk 9:1; Lk 9:27: "Truly I tell you, there are some standing here who will not taste death before they see the Son of Man coming in his kingdom, "and Mt 24:34; Mk 13:30; Lk 21:32: "Truly, I tell you, this generation will not pass away until all these things have taken place." Also, Mt 23:36; Lk 11:50 speaks of the judgment coming on the Jews in *"this generation."*[14]

It may appear that the Gospel writers were poor predictors. They were likely commenting on the times, including the Temple's destruction in 70 CE and the Romans' persecution. Within the Gospels, we also have the understanding that *But of the hour no one knows, neither the angels of heaven, nor the Son, but the Father alone"* can say when the

---

[14] Ibid, 295.

end will come (Mt 24:36; Mk 13:32). Jesus, it can be assumed, living in those times of Roman occupation, would have a sense of urgency regarding the judgment on the people of God (Israelites) and the destruction of the Temple. Moreover, why does Jesus take the time to prepare those who are to follow him? The Apostles of Jesus and other disciples are commissioned to go into the world as witnesses. The disciples are told they will have to endure hardship and suffering at the hands of their enemies. Yet the notice is clear; without their witness, Jesus' message cannot survive. Speculation is insignificant to the living of the Word of God and going out teaching and preaching, which is best expressed in "Great Commissioning" (Mt 28:18-20):

> *Then Jesus approached and said to them, "All power in heaven and on earth has been given to me. Go, therefore, and make disciples of all nations, baptizing them in the name of the Father, and of the Son, and of the Holy Spirit, teaching them to observe all that I have commanded you. And behold, I am with you always, until the end of the age."*

The disciples are being exhorted to teach the moral lesson found in Jesus' message, principally that of the Sermon on the Mount (Mt 5–7). The commandments of Jesus are the standard of Christian conduct. It is not the Mosaic law as such, even though some of the Mosaic commandments have now been invested with Jesus' authority. *Behold, I am with you always: the promise of Jesus' real though invisible presence echoes Emmanuel's name* (God with us) given to him in Matthew's infancy narrative.

Summary

This chapter has discussed various cultural influences that helped shape how Christianity understands how Christ is fulfilling the Old Testament prophesies and the fullness of the truth that is not available in other religions. Virtually all world religions include the universal moral laws such as the Golden Rule: humility, charity, and honesty. Paul's teaching differentiates Christianity through God's intervention in the world by the Incarnation and the Holy Spirit. God is present in the form of the Trinity. The death and resurrection of Jesus enable God's salvation for humanity. The presence of the Holy Spirit is evidence of God's continuing presence in the world. The Gospel writers also describe Jesus as the key to salvation.

The next chapter will deal with the controversial topic of miracles. I will then move into a discussion of virtuous living before expanding to how individuals and organizations can exhibit virtue. I choose to discuss miracles first because we often confuse faith with superstitious beliefs about how God intervenes in human life. Miracles are often seen as evidence of God's favoring of particular individuals. They are seen as a reward for faith. I want to address this issue directly before a discussion of virtuous living.

Suggested Reading

What Paul Meant by Gary Wills gives a clear, easy-to-read understanding of Paul's views, which are so crucial to the development of Christian thinking both in the early Church and right on to this day.

Chapter Five

Let's Talk about Miracles

But so that you may know that the Son of Man has authority on earth to forgive sins"—then He said to the paralyzed man, "Get up, pick up your stretcher and go home." And he got up and went home. But when the crowds saw this, they were awestruck, and they glorified God, who had given such authority to men. (Matthew 9:6-8)

To this point in the book, I have referenced several scriptural commentaries. This approach was to give the reader an idea of how I have arrived at my assumptions. A discussion of miracles may seem out of place because I have previously stated that it was Jesus' message that is the enduring legacy of His ministry. Talking about miracles seems to be inconsistent with that idea. Unfortunately, my justification is that all too many of us have transactional relationships with God that depend on prayers being answered in precisely the way we want for us to believe. Jesus' message is lost if we base faith on a promise that God will materially bless us or grant our "wish." I intend to discuss this idea of a transactional relationship with God as being a disordered way of expressing one's faith.

A second reason for introducing a chapter on miracles is that I have seen within my work and reports from providers about patient/family requests for treatment judged to be non-beneficial and even harmful. They make these requests because they are "hoping for a miracle." Although it is difficult to fault their sense of urgency, I find it particularly important to discuss this because "holding out for a miracle" often results in the patient, family, and even provider avoiding taking action to benefit the patient. Therefore, an understanding of miracles is supportive of all parties involved in the case of a life-limiting illness. In a later chapter, I will discuss the importance of informed consent. Knowledge about the nature and purpose of miracles is crucial to being able to make informed decisions.

Over the last 30+ years, I have engaged in independent reading, seminars, retreats, and over a thousand sermons. I am a graduate of the Aquinas Institute of Theology in the Master of Arts in Health Care Ministry program. I also completed the Graduate Certificate in Biblical Studies program. I am now completing the Master of Arts in Theology also at the Aquinas Institute of Theology. I intend to use the information that I have accumulated over the years and integrate it into a meaningful discussion concerning how we can use the principles of Christianity to "live as long as we can, as well as we can." I want to continue the conversation by discussing the idea of miracles. Miracles are difficult for us in the Western world to accept, considering our belief that nature's laws are unchallengeable. Yet, when we read the Bible stories of miracles, we must remember that the audience for whom the episodes are directed sees the world from a very different perspective. For them, the world was a strange and mysterious place where spirits, good and evil, had incredible control.

Reginald Fuller shows how, in Matthew 11:4-6, Jesus reveals his healing miracles' real meaning. Jesus' oblique answer to John's disciples was, *Go and tell John what you see: the blind regain their sight, the lame walk, lepers are cleansed, the deaf hear, the dead are raised, and the poor have the good news proclaimed to them.* Jesus does not say that He is doing these mighty deeds. Instead, it is Jesus affirming that his miracles are works of God wrought through him. Fuller says Jesus never directly says he is the source of the miracles.[1] Often observers cite the miracles of Jesus as evidence of his divinity. Fuller disagrees that this is the way the Bible uses them. "They are not proofs but signs—signs for those who have eyes to see and ears to hear."[2] They are signs of God's presence through the Incarnation.

---

[1] Reginald H and Alfred Daniel Westberg, *Preaching the Lectionary: The Word of God for the Church Today.* (Collegeville, MN: Liturgical Press, 2006), 9.

[2] Ibid.

C.S. Lewis, one of the most famous writers of all time and a devout Christian, had much to say about miracles. Walter Hooper, in his book *C.S Lewis, Companion and Guide*, says:

"The traditional Christian view of miracles was stated by St Athanasius (c. 296 – 373) in the eighteenth section of his famous De Incarnatione..." Our LORD took a body like to ours and lived as a man in order that those who had refused to recognize him in His superintendence and captaincy of the whole universe might come to recognize from the works, he did here below in the body that what dwelled in this body was the Word of God.' And this, said Lewis, 'accords exactly with Christ's own account of his miracles: "The Son can do nothing of himself, but what he seeth the Father do." Following in the same tradition, St. Thomas Aquinas (c. 1225 – 74) said, 'those happenings are properly called miraculous which a divine agency does outside the commonly observed order of things.' By the time Lewis turned his mind to miracles, most theologians had stopped believing in the same way as Athanasius and Aquinas. The belief in the improbability of miracles was mainly a result of the rise of modern science in the seventeenth and eighteenth centuries, which increasingly saw the world as a closed system subject to the laws of Nature. Lewis himself, in his atheist years, had learned much of his skepticism from David Hume's famous Essay on Miracles (1748) and the writings of philosophers such as G.W.F. Hegel, who identified God with the Law of Nature. Lewis knew from the beginning that a defense of the miracles recorded in the New Testament would have to begin with a philosophical attack on unbelief."[3]

My intention is to view the idea of miracles from a perspective that tries to harmonize a faith in a higher power (which I define as belief and trust in the teachings of Jesus) and our understanding of scientific (physical science) knowledge. I want to help the reader understand our relationship with God to be one of faith and trust, rather than an if/then transaction. I will endeavor to show that by accepting God's divine plan, we are not eliminating hope. Instead, as stated earlier, hope allows us to endure suffering and, in fact, aids us in living a life and a passion for creating a just world here and now. Hope is not expecting an unrealistic result as a reward for a life well-lived. Hope is the understanding of the ultimate ability to know God in the fullest sense of the word.

---

[3] Walter Hooper, *C.S. Lewis: The Companion and Guide,* (San Francisco, CA: HarperSanFrancisco, 1996), 342-3343.

I was on retreat with some of the men I referred to earlier. Each of us was tasked with suggesting a topic for discussion during the retreat. I choose to discuss miracles, specifically, do miracles still happen? During the discussion, one of the participants made a statement that, while humorous, is altogether too often true. He jokingly said, "A miracle is a result of good fortune which happens to me or my family and is not expected." This comment was an expression of how lightly we use the term miracle. We use the word miracle to characterize any beneficial event that is statistically unlikely but not contrary to nature's laws, such as surviving a natural disaster or only a "wonderful" occurrence, such as a birth. Other such miracles we nominate are the survival of an illness diagnosed as terminal, escaping a life-threatening situation, a game-winning home-run, or "beating the odds," such as winning the lottery.

Here are two ways to describe miracles. A miracle is an event that the forces of nature—including the natural powers of man—cannot of themselves produce, which must be referred to as a supernatural agency.[4] We can also say a miracle is a divine operation that transcends what is normally perceived as natural law; it cannot be explained on any expected basis. C.S. Lewis talks of two general classifications for miracles: miracles of Old Creation and miracles

---

[4] George P. Fisher, *Manual of Christian Evidences* (New York, NY: Charles Scribner's Sons, 1894), 9.

of New Creation.[5] The Old Creation type interacts with the real world. This type of miracle reproduces operations we have already seen on a larger scale but does so in a magnified way with a much more immediate result. For instance, Jesus' curing is the stimulation of natural processes; he can promote nature to remove hindrances from affecting a cure. Old Creation miracles are ones in which we see divine intervention influence something that is not unnatural within nature. For example, we can postulate that healing results from God's providence working through the caregiver's technology and personal involvement. If God is the creator of all, then one can also believe that miracles constitute an intervention within nature. A miracle is the activity of God, and its result follows the laws of nature. Old Creation miracles deal with fertility, healing, destruction, and power over nature. For instance, turning water into wine is a natural process in which he accelerates the fermentation process to demonstrate His love and obedience, and compassion for the bride and groom. When Jesus heals, he can direct the self-correcting nature of a person's own body. Jesus can harness the divine power within all of us due to our being made in God's image and likeness.

The New Creation offers the promise of a new state of being, a glorification of the state to reflect a perfecting of

---

[5] C. S. Lewis, *Miracles: A Preliminary Study* (San Francisco: HarperOne, 2001). 221-231.

our spiritual state. New Creation miracles give us a glimpse of things that have not yet been; they look into the future. New Creation focuses on God's action still to come. Walking on water, raising the dead, the Transfiguration, the Resurrection, and Ascension are examples of miracles that foreshadow future events. New Creation miracles point to humans' ultimate destiny. They point us to a new state of affairs where there will be a perfect expression of oneness with God.

The Catechism of the Catholic Church declares:

Because of his transcendence, God cannot be seen as he is, unless he himself opens up his mystery to man's immediate contemplation and gives him the capacity for it. The Church calls this contemplation of God in his heavenly glory "the *beatific vision*."

How great will your glory and happiness be, to be allowed to see God, to be honored with sharing the joy of salvation and eternal light with Christ your LORD and God, . . . to delight in the joy of immortality in the Kingdom of heaven with the righteous and God's friends. (St. Cyprian) (*CCC* 1028)

The classification of miracles, in my opinion, places greater significance on the miracles of the New Creation as it points to the completion of humans' journey to full communion with God. All the great religions speak of some manner of perfection, be it nirvana or paradise, where all your desires are satisfied. Yet, this is the state that many, and particularly American Christians, most actively try to avoid.

I am reminded of the story of the preacher who asks his congregation to "raise your hand if you want to go to heaven." Of course, all the people respond in the affirmative. He then follows up with a second question: "How about right now?" All hands go down! Americans and other Western thinking people appear to have an ambivalence about their view of the hereafter. While we are taught to look forward to being one with our maker, we act in such a way to avoid such a meeting without regard to cost or quality of life. We pray for miracles, which are almost exclusively Old Creation. That is, we look for healing (physical) or make other petitions that give us confidence that God has the "power to do whatever; nothing is impossible." Our prayers tend to petition, asking for supernatural intervention in our human world.

There are five broad categories of miracles to which our petitions are directed. First, we seek miracles that involve a temporary and location-specific suspension of laws regulating nature. For instance, Jesus walked upon the waters of the Sea of Galilee (Jn 6:16-21). We ask God to change the course of tornadoes, bring or stop the rain, and any number of other suspensions of the laws of nature that inconvenience us. Jesus' stories concerning the control of nature hold a deeper meaning than the physical act, which is observed. For example, let us take Jesus' calming a ferocious storm on the Sea of Galilee (Mk 4:35-41; Mt 8:23-27; Lk 8:22-25). This type of event is a miracle of Old Creation as it deals with something that happens regularly in nature.

I can speak with some authority on how this story may have developed. During my trip to Galilee, I had the opportunity to take a boat ride on the lake. That afternoon the lake was very calm and provided an enjoyable experience. A few hours later, when it was just beginning to get dark, my wife and I were sitting outside on the lawn at our hotel, which overlooked the lake. Suddenly, an enormous wind came up, which created large waves and whitecaps on the lake. This storm lasted for no more than 5 minutes (if that long), and then the lake was again calm. I am told such events are not uncommon due to the area's topography since the lake is surrounded by mountains and below sea level. The wind can "kick-up" and blow through the lake valley furiously. The disciples were undoubtedly aware of such phenomena. Then why do the synoptic writers all include this story?

The story demonstrates Jesus' humanity. He was tired and needed rest. The apostles' lack of faith reminds us that even those who lived and walked with Jesus saw his miracles and heard his message still found it challenging to be 100 percent faith-filled all the time. In that way, the disciples were a lot like us. However, their lack of faith was re-buked—and, by extension, so is ours. If Jesus was able to rescue the apostles from the storm, He could save us from the storms of everyday life: sickness, job loss, marriage problems, and even the sting of death (1 Cor 15:55). The significance of the storm's taming, it seems, has more to do with the peace we can have in sorrow or anxiety. It express-es the ability to turn the darkness of despair into the sun-shine of eternal life. During that storm, Jesus' presence in the boat is a reminder to us that he is ever-present to share our experience.

Second, we look for signs that involve the healing of man's physical body. The Gospels give us over 20 examples of Jesus' healing, including multiple instances of action that included the blind, paralyzed, and lepers. He also healed people of other orthopedic infirmities (dropsy and withered hand) as well as the Centurion's servant (Mt 8:5-13; Lk 7:1-10; Jn 4:46-54). Ironically, Jesus tells us that his main task is to preach and teach. He did not want to be seen as a "Da-vidic" king or warrior. That is why he so often asked those around him not to speak of his action. His healing acts are signs of compassion and mercy rather than power. The per-formance of healing provides proof that Jesus has a special relationship with God. It was believed that healing was ex-clusively a divine power restricted to very few Priestly clas-ses in Jesus' time. Jesus' healing confirmed that his power came from a divine source. His healing acts impressed the people, yet they did not appear to be sufficient to retain followers over the long run. Even his disciples deserted him at the end. They were only to be convinced by the resurrection, which is a Miracle of the New Age.

Third, signs were demonstrating divine power over death. Lazarus, dead for four days, was raised (Jn 11:43-44). The act of resuscitating Lazarus foreshadowed Christ's own power over death. Yet, while he brought Lazarus back to life, this did not give Lazarus everlasting life. Everlasting life is the product of the resurrection of Christ, which is a miracle of New Creation and the very foundation of the Christian system (1 Cor 15:16-19).

Fourth, many of the New Testament age wonders had to do with the expulsion of demons that had entered human bodies. Several instances of those possessed by demons are depicted in the New Testament. They include in Mark 1:21-28, the man with an unclean spirit in the synagogue at Capernaum; 5:1-20, the demoniac with a legion of unclean spirits among the tombs in Gerasene; 7:24-30, the daughter of the Syrophoenician woman possessed by an unclean spirit or demon; 9:14-29, the boy with the dumb spirit, often called the epileptic boy. Matthew and Luke use some of the same stories. They also mention Jesus casting a demon out in Matthew 8:28-34 and 12:22-32. Luke contains the healing of the Gerasene demoniac in 8:26-39. In the first century, demons were considered the root cause of all evil. Scripture describes demons resulting from the fall of some angels. Certain Scriptures tell that Satan fell from heaven and other angelic beings shared in Satan's fall and became evil. In particular, Ezekiel 28:11-19 tells the story of a creature of God who becomes so impressed with himself that he begins to desire the place of honor and power that is God's alone. His name was changed from Lucifer (Morning Star) to Satan (Adversary), and he, along with his followers, was banished from heaven, taking up residence on earth where they are a constant cause of problems for humankind.

In Jesus' time, demons were ubiquitous and thought to cause illness and great mischief in the world. We need only look at the Gerasene demon-possessed man's story that appears in all three synoptic gospels. With some variation (Matthew's version has two demon-possessed men), we are offered a quite familiar situation to the people of Palestine. We have Jesus crossing the Sea of Galilee and landing in an area where many limestone caves were used for burial places. I have seen this area and can attest to how weird such a situation might appear at night. This period is also a time that is right for the appearance of demons. The man is very disturbed, sometimes speaking in the singular as if speaking for himself and speaking in the plural as if it is the demons speaking. His possession's intensity is attested to because he had to make more than one attempt to rid him of the demons. Jesus first used his customary authoritative order for the demon to come out, which was not successful. Next, he demanded the demon to identify itself by name. The understanding of the time was that knowing the name gave one power over the demon. Then Jesus offered tangible proof by driving the demons into a herd of swine. This act assured the man that the demon(s) were driven out.

Commentators often make a great deal about the demon's name, Legion, and having the demons driven into the unclean animals. They opine that this story is much about opposition to Roman rule (Galilee was a hotbed of rebellion). For my part, I think the story is a demonstration of Jesus' understanding that for the man to be healed, he had to be shown that Jesus had the power to overcome the demons. Jesus understood the mind of the people regarding the fear of spirits and how control could be demonstrated. The name Legion gives us a clue that the man may have had a traumatic event involving conflict with the Romans. He may have had what we term Post Traumatic Stress Disorder. Jesus' calling out the demon's name probably resulted in the man's yelling out and thereby frightening the herd of swine. For our purposes, Jesus' demonstration of mercy toward the man is the most significant aspect of the story. Ironically, the people of the area reacted to Jesus' act by asking him to leave. Not only had he run the swine off, but they were also fearful of his power over the spirit world. Again, this is an example of Jesus' action having a result that we, as 21st-century people, do not fully comprehend. We like to see Jesus' action as an expression of his power over Satan. Jesus showed the value and worth of even the most despicable people in his time. Acknowledging each person's dignity leads me to discuss the use of miracles by "healers" today.

I find it ironic that so many so-called "faith healers" and fundamentalist preachers continue to act as though demons cause illness and tragedy. They seem to insist that a person become redeemed before any healing can take place. There is a fundamental belief that the person has little value or worth until they make a public pronouncement of accepting Jesus. I find this difficult to harmonize with Jesus' displays of mercy and compassion. Although scripture suggests that faith is a fundamental ingredient in healing, Jesus does not condemn but uses the recovery to affirm the person's worth. Jesus' action allows the demoniac to again come into full communion with their community. I often find we use our religious convictions on people instead of with and for people in their time of distress. Jesus was present for people; he invited them to be part of a loving family of believers to experience "the kingdom of God here on earth."

Fifth, we see the manipulation of natural material such as Christ's turning water into wine (Jn 2:1-11) and multiplying a boy's loaves and fishes so that thousands were fed (Jn 6:1-14). When we explore these stories, we must keep in mind that John and the synoptic writers often spoke metaphorically. These writers were not interested in constructing a literal historical account. Instead, they aimed to reveal the truth of Jesus in a way that has meaning for all ages. The writers used the story to convey a message that went beyond a mere recitation of facts. By looking at the wedding story at Canaan, we can see how the writer uses this story to set the stage for Jesus' sacrifice. Let's take some of the story elements and "drill down" to demonstrate what I mean.

John 2:1 begins: *On the third day, there was a wedding in Cana of Galilee, and the mother of Jesus was there.* Those who have spent time reading the Bible appreciate the significance of numbers like 3, 7, and 40 as symbolic rather than literal. The fact that this event occurred on the third day is a way of saying, "something big is going to happen." The marriage feast is symbolic of joy that accompanies the coming of God. Jesus is requested to do something, and he politely replies, *My hour has not yet come* (Jn 2:4). Nevertheless, Jesus is obedient and demonstrates this obedience (to God) by providing a "sign" of that which is to come.

His miracle includes the use of the jars of ritual purification used at the wedding in our story. The pots are enormous (six jars of 20 to 30 gallons), thus magnifying the significance of the action Jesus is about to undertake. Jesus' turning the water to wine is figurative of his blood (symbolized in the Last Supper by the wine) as the real source of purification. It is a foreshadowing of the crucifixion. The sign which John and only John describes reveals to us Jesus' ultimate journey. The story of changing water to wine pales compared with the actual revealed truth of Christ's sacrifice for our sake.

The stories of the feeding of large groups of people in Matthew 15:32-16:10 and Mark 8:1-9 (4000) and John 6:5-15 and Luke 9:12-17 (5000) speak to Jesus 'demonstration of the importance of the bread of life that he represents. These stories are representative of Jesus' compassion for the people. It is also a story that ties the Old Testament story of God's providing manna for the Israelites in the desert in Exodus 16:1-36. The story connects to the story of Elisha in 2 Kings. Elisha tells his servant to feed the people gathered there, although there was not enough food for the hundred men. One of the men said, *How can I set this before a hundred men* (2 Kings 4:42–43). In the end, however, the men not only had enough to eat, but *they ate and had some left* (2 Kings 4:44). These stories demonstrate God's generosity as more than enough is provided. The story symbolizes Jesus' divinity through his ability to multiply the available resources and his compassion.

The feeding of large groups of people is the only story (albeit with slight variations) described in all four gospels. It is a story in which Jesus uses his disciples to serve rather than making the food just appear. *He gave . . . to his disciples to distribute to the people* (Mk 6:41). The disciples were thus placed in a position of having total trust in what Jesus was instructing them to do. The message is that we are to trust that God will meet our needs. This action is not a trust that is dependent on a transactional relationship with God. What we are being told is that if we trust without reservation, God will provide. This understanding is different from the transactional way in which we often approach our relationship with God. That is, if you do this for me, then I will do it for you. The story of the feeding of the masses tells us that we are cared for and protected if we trust.

How do we know it is a miracle?

When Jesus performed signs (miracles), even his enemies did not deny the effect of such; they merely attempted to attribute his power to some other source (e.g., Beelzebub, the prince of demons, Mt 12:24). The Jewish community leaders did not doubt that Peter and John had performed a notable miracle when they healed the lame man at the temple; instead, they sought to mute the sign's impact by threats of violence (Acts 4:14).

Wayne Jackson, an evangelical, Protestant theologian, gives us descriptions of the characteristics of miracles.[6] Miracles always have a worthy motive. Though Jesus' miracles established the validity of his claim of being the Son of

---

[6] Wayne Jackson, "What Does the Bible Say About Miracles?" *Christian Courier* (Christian Courier, 2019), online at https://www.christiancourier.com/articles/5-what-does-the-bible-say-about-miracles.

God, that designation was not assumed out of personal interest. Instead, his action was motivated by a love for humans and a clear demonstration of mercy and compassion. Christ and his disciples did not perform wonders in the first century to enhance themselves financially. They were unlike the wealthy "faith healers" of today. When Peter encountered the lame man of Acts 3, he had no money (v. 6). Generally, the Bible era's miracles were done in the presence of many credible witnesses, even hostile observers. When the LORD multiplied the loaves and fishes, possibly some 10 thousand or more people were present (Jn 6:10). Genuine miracles were not slow, progressive processes. They produced instantaneous effects. For example, Bartimaeus *immediately received his sight and followed him on his way* (Mk 10:52). At Peter's curing of the disabled beggar immediately, his feet and *ankle grew strong* (Acts 3:7). In the New Testament, one never reads such statements as this: "Jesus prayed for him, and within three weeks, he was cured."

Real miracles must be subject to sense perception. The water that Jesus turned into wine could be tasted (Jn 2:9); Thomas could feel the prints in the hands of the resurrected Christ (Jn 20:27), and the restored ear of the high priest's servant could be seen (Lk 22:51). C.S. Lewis uses the word "miracle" to mean interference with nature by a supernatural power.[7] By this, he says there must be no possible way to explain the miracle naturally.

For instance, I have a heart arrhythmia that causes premature ventricular contractions (PVCs). PVCs are extra, abnormal heartbeats that begin in one of your heart's two lower pumping chambers (ventricles). These extra beats disrupt your regular heart rhythm, sometimes causing you to feel a flip-flop or skipped beat in your chest. Frequent PVCs can sap your energy and be quite debilitating. The treatment for a person such as me who has had many such episodes is called an ablation. The American Heart Association describes ablation as a procedure that uses radiofrequency energy (like microwave heat) to destroy a small heart tissue area causing rapid and irregular heartbeats.[8] Destroying this tissue helps restore the heart's regular rhythm. People who undergo such a procedure will feel immediate relief and restoration. I have heard people call this procedure (as well as many other medical procedures) a miracle. Yet, what occurs is easily explainable in natural terms. If one is as fortunate as I was, the procedure will be done in a hospital that understands the healing presence of

---

[7] Lewis, 12.

[8] "Ablation for Arrhythmias," *American Heart Association*, accessed February 22, 2021, https://www.heart.org/en/health-topics/arrhythmia/prevention--treatment-of-arrhythmia/ablation-for-arrhythmias.

Jesus in giving confidence to the patient and the caregiver. This result does not qualify as a miracle since the process can be explained naturally. Yet, I often have heard people call such a procedure a miracle.

Some commentators have used "common sense" explanations in discussing Jesus' miracles. The multitudes' feeding may simply have been the crowds deciding to share the food they have brought along for the day (I do not subscribe to this explanation). The storm on the Sea of Galilee is a regular occurrence, a natural phenomenon in which Jesus' presence brought comfort. Nevertheless, some miracles defy explanation. For instance, it cannot be argued that the blind man of John 9:1 was psychosomatically afflicted, for the gentleman had been in that condition since birth. The woman's healing with blood flow (Mk 5:25; Mt 9:20; Lk 8:43) came only after many physicians' efforts were unsuccessful. How can a perfectly restored ear previously amputated be explained by current processes (Lk 22:50-51)? We can see an underlying message in each of these miracle stories but must acknowledge that natural causes cannot explain some of these incidents.

Do miracles still occur?

I believe that part of a Christian faith tradition would have no problem accepting most, if not all, the stories of miracles in the Bible as believable. They could believe even

if they did not occur in some exact factual scenario presented in the text. That is, some are primarily concerned with
the writer's meaning. They use a historical/contextual approach to Scripture study to look at who wrote the text and
when it was completed? They ask questions like, what is the
literary genre (form criticism)? What is the socio-historical
context which asks questions such as?

- If the story claims to be historical, what happened?
- What social, historical, or cultural information can
  be gleaned from the text?
- What is background information necessary to understand the text better?
- What was lifelike for the ordinary people, not just
  the ruling elites?

Within these ways of studying Scripture, we find the
common denominator identifying Jesus' action to confirm
the Incarnate Word: God made human. Therefore, the supernatural gifts had as their design the establishment of
Christ's credibility and that of his spokespersons. Ultimately, the desire was to validate their message, namely that Jesus Christ is the Son of God. A supernatural display of divine power is not an arguable proposition; it is a dramatic,
verifiable fact. Miracles either happen, or they don't.

Do most of those things we proclaim as miracles meet the criteria I have established above? I would submit that most do not. Does that mean that miracles do not occur today? Two essential features of the requirements for being deemed a miracle are immediacy and the absence of any mediating variable (medical intervention, for instance). These characteristics are often absent in those healing miracles that we declare have happened. A third factor, abiding purpose, is also frequently missing. The act we label as a miracle is for a single episode and benefit. The underlying message of mercy and compassion for all is lost in the interest of the one. However, we should not deny that miracles of healing do occur; they merely occur with much less frequency than we think. By calling every unusual event a miracle, we lose the meaning and purpose of those things that genuinely are miracles.

St. Thomas teaches: "Those effects are rightly to be termed miracles which are wrought by Divine power apart from the order usually observed in nature" (Contra Gent., III, cii), and they are apart from the natural order because they are "beyond the order or laws of the whole created nature" (ST- I, Q. cii, a. 4).[9] Miracles result from immediate intervention by a divine source (most often Jesus) or through a representative who is recognized to be an agent

---

[9] Gerald O'Collins and Edward G. Farrugia, A Concise Dictionary of Theology, (New York: Paulist Press, 2000), 160.

of God. A miracle must be worthy of the holiness, goodness, and justice of God and conducive to the true good of
men. Miracles are not performed to repair physical defects
in God's creation, nor are they intended to produce or create disorder and discord. Miracles do not contain any element that is wicked, ridiculous, useless, or insignificant. A
miracle is not intended to be contrary or opposed to nature:
its impact demonstrates God's mercy and love for his creatures. Miracles do not extend the life beyond reasonable
expectations based on the age and condition of the individual. Miracles are not the product of a bargain with God or a
payoff for living a righteous life.

My conclusion is that we, as humans, have trivialized
miracles by labeling what may be good fortune or a triumph of human intellect (a gift from God) as a miracle.
This action makes us immune to the profound impact real
miracles can offer. By seeing only the physical change, we
often miss the idea that we have been freed from what
keeps us from being whole. My answer to the question, do
miracles still occur, is yes. I answer in the affirmative with
the provision that we must be cautious in claiming that
something is a miracle. A simple definition of what can be
called a miracle is found in O'Collins and Farrugia's: *A
Concise Dictionary of Theology.*

[A miracle) is an event caused by special divine action
that does not follow the normal laws of nature and car-

ries a religious message for people now and later. Far from being mere astonishing prodigies (rare events), miracles are saving and revealing signs from God (Jn 2:11, 18, 23; 12:18, 37). The Synoptic Gospels (Mt 4:23; 8:5-17; 11:5, 21; Mk 8:22-26; Lk 13:32; Acts 2:22 witness to Jesus' miracles, which were tied in with his powerful proclamation of God's final kingdom.[10]

Miracles are more than merely unexplainable events. Nor are they only exhibitions of supernatural power. Miracles are part of the plan of salvation. The Economy of Salvation deals with God's creation and management of the world, notably his plan of salvation that is to be facilitated through the Church's action. Miracles are, therefore, an affirmation of the message that Christ brings to the world. They are part of the elements and resources revealed by God as necessary for the sake of humanity's salvation through revelation and messages given, primarily through the person of Jesus Christ. The salvation economy is further made up of Christ's being sacrificed on the cross, his resurrection, the gift of the Holy Spirit to humanity, the Church, and the sacraments. Miracles are a vital part of the whole divine Economy of Salvation, not something that exists solely outside the entirety of the plan of salvation.

---

[10] "Miracle," *Catholic Answers* (Catholic Answers, February 22, 2019), https://www.catholic.com/encyclopedia/miracle.

Summary

All too often, we define miracles in ways that trivialize the real significance of Jesus' demonstration of mercy and compassion. Miracles have specifically defined characteristics that signify that something extraordinary and beyond human explanation has occurred. Miracles do happen, but they are not a reward or sign that one is favored over another. Miracles are not merely unusual events with no apparent explanation. Miracles are an intervention in nature that has a causal link back to God. A miracle brings people into God's kingdom by demonstrating the presence of a loving Father for whom all things were possible.

More important, for caregivers and those affected by a life-limiting illness, there is a frequent inclination to bargain for more time by "holding out for a miracle." The focus becomes the survival of the physical being. Such actions are often not only not beneficial, but they can also be harmful. Moreover, it distracts all the parties from embracing the types of actions that provide comfort, support, and spiritual nourishment for all involved.

Suggested Reading

Miracles, by C.S. Lewis, is a concise explanation of miracles as a witness of God's exceptional personal involvement in his creation. It is a well-written confirmation of his understanding of miracles.

The Spirituality of Mark: Responding to God, written by Southern Baptist theologian Mitzi Minor has a good discussion of faith, spirituality, and its relationship to miracles.

Chapter Six

The Nature of a Virtuous Life

Finally, brothers, whatever is true,
whatever is honorable,
whatever is just, whatever is pure,
whatever is lovely, whatever is gracious,
if there is any excellence
and if there is anything worthy of praise
think about these things. (Philippians 4:8-9)

A discussion of virtuous living must begin with an enumeration of the virtues seen as essential to right living. The cardinal virtues are prudence, justice, fortitude, and temperance. Anyone can practice these behaviors. They form the basis of natural morality that governs developed societies. They are logical rules that advance common-sense guidelines for living responsibly with fellow human beings and represent the values Christians are directed to use in their interactions. The second set of virtues are theological virtues. These are gifts of grace from God. Theological virtues are given to us freely, not through any action on our part, and we are free, but not required, to accept and use them. These are the virtues by which humans relate to God: faith, hope, and charity (love). While these terms have ordinary secular meaning, they take a unique sense when talking about human relationships and God.

This section of the book deals with specific thoughts concerning how one can live life to prepare for God's kingdom. It will also provide some examples of extraordinary and ordinary people who have lived remarkably virtuous lives.

St. Augustine believed that it is the proposition of faith that animates our relationship with God. For Christians, this faith and belief in the power of God is the very foundation of our understanding of God's eternal plan for humanity. He acknowledged the importance of scientific knowledge to assist us in understanding the world God created. Yet, the final authority was held to interpret God's word as revealed through the Church to him. Later, Thomas Aquinas introduced the idea that God is revealed to us through common intelligence, fed by our five senses. Aquinas moved Christianity from the mystical, purely spiritual side to something that humans could come to understand, albeit incompletely, through reason. Aquinas held that our faith in eternal salvation shows that we have theological truths that exceed human rights. In an article entitled *Philosophy for Beginners: The Theology of Death*, Fr. Brian Mullady tells us:

St. Thomas Aquinas is very clear about the nature of death. He says: "The necessity of dying for Man is partly from nature and partly from sin." Death due to nature is caused by the contrary elements of the body. Every material element in the body is composed of both active and passive elements held together in a tenuous connection. From the point of view of these elements, death is natural. Nor is there any power in the material elements themselves or in the soul to keep my body or any body from death. From the point of view of the body, then Man is mortal and doomed to die.[1]

Mullady explains that although the body is composed of transient matter, humans also have a soul that gives us form. Form, in its most simple terms, is that which we become. Mullady says, "The form of Man is his reasoning soul, which is immortal, wherefore death is not natural to Man from this form or this soul."[2] For Aquinas, humans' form or soul is not limited by the matter's restrictions, including the human body. Through being formed, humans can accept salvation, which is offered without requiring a return benefit. For Aquinas, death is both painful and full of sorrow as a penalty for sin. Nevertheless, because we can

---

[1] Brian Mullady, *Philosophy for Beginners: The Theology of Death*, http://ccgaction.org/spiritual_life/theologyofdeath

[2] Ibid.

be formed, we can have a complete relationship with God that transcends the matter's natural end.

John Cardinal Henry Newman built on human ability to come into a complete relationship with God comparing two forms of assent that we use, especially in dealing with death.[3] One type of assent is what he calls notional, in which I apply only abstract reasoning that does not involve me in a personal way. With notional assent, I can put death out of my mind; yes, it happens to all of us, but it is not something to worry about now. Real assent is an intensely personal acknowledgment that brings me "face to face" with my relationship with others and, more importantly, my relationship with God.[4]

Notional assent results in a simple acknowledgment of the inevitability of death, yet it does not stir me to action. Real assent provokes a response to rectify those things about my life that cause me shame or which have harmed others. It is the point where I admit my sinfulness and come to recognize that it is through the power of God that I am offered salvation. For Newman, it is not fear that brings one to real assent. Instead, it allows us to use the intellectual understanding we have of God as part of our discernment

---

[3] John F. Crosby, "The Personalism of John Henry Newman," *The Catholic Thing* (Sept. 14, 2019). https://thecatholicthing.org/2019/09/14/the-personalism-of-john-henry-newman/

[4] Ibid.

process to come to an intensely personal relationship with God. We can then make what I term an "informed assent" commitment to a relationship with God. John F. Crosby says Newman wants to release the transformative power of the truth we already acknowledge. Real assent exists in the most profound personal reality. With notional assent, I may objectively accept my coming death, whereas, with real assent, I tremble at the thought of it. Real assent is personal, unlike subjectivism, which sees no objective truth.[5] Crosby adds that Newman thinks that this critical distinction is also found in our relation to God. He states that Newman believes one can know God by way of what he calls the "theological intellect," which is to know him notionally. It is through "religious imagination" that I come to know him.[6] Newman explains religious imagination as "the experience of being morally obliged, or in the experience of being ashamed because of some wrong I have done, I encounter the living God in my conscience, I am in his presence. I experience my creaturehood and his sovereignty."[7]

Newman's religious imagination is not the relativism so prevalent in post-modern thinking where there is no external or objective truth. This kind of thinking roots back to the 18th and 19th centuries when philosophers like David

---

[5] Ibid.

[6] Ibid.

[7] Ibid.

Hume and Immanuel Kant sought to prove that religious truth lay outside the scope of human understanding and could not be known with certainty. Newman questions whether conscience is rooted in some form of transcendent moral law or not. For Newman, it is the transcendent moral law of which he writes:

> He became Creator, he implanted this Law, which is himself, in the intelligence of all his rational creatures. The Divine Law, then, is the rule of ethical truth, the standard of right and wrong, a sovereign, irreversible, absolute authority in the presence of men and Angels.[8]

When Newman talks about the law, he is talking about human conscience. Because our conscience comes from our Creator, it also has both rights and responsibilities derived from the same source. That source is God and his law by which he has ordered the world. In a relativist world, it is only rights that seem to count. This concept is different from how we ordinarily speak of conscience. It is founded on the doctrine that conscience is God's voice, rather than considering it to be created by humans. Christians' highest

---

[8] Admin, "Conscience, Newman, and the Pope." *The Catholic Thing* (Sept. 18, 2015, https://www.thecatholicthing.org/2015/02/25/conscience-newman-pope/.

responsibility is to know God and embrace the divine truth derived through a relationship with Christ.

I contend that living a virtuous life is hinged on an internal moral compass that is pointed to the "true north" of God's revealed truth. All too often, the conscience for the person of faith, and particularly Christians, is seen as a moral straitjacket that allows no freedom of choice. Freedom is considered to be the ability "to ignore a Lawgiver and Judge, to be independent of unseen obligations."[9] Freedom with only rights and no obligations is a relativistic view not shared by Christians. The *Catholic Church's Catechism* deals with freedom in Part Three, "Life in Christ," Article 3, "Man's Freedom."

> <u>**1730**</u> God created man a rational being, conferring on him the dignity of a person who can initiate and control his own actions. "God willed that man should be 'left in the hand of his own counsel,' so that he might of his own accord seek his Creator and freely attain his full and blessed perfection by cleaving to him." Man is rational and therefore, like God; he is created with free will and is master over his acts.

---

[9] Servais Théodore Pinckaers, *Morality: The Catholic View*, trans. Michael Sherwin (South Bend, IN: St. Augustine's Press, 2001), 78.

The *Catechism* goes on to explain freedom as:

> **1731** Freedom is the power, rooted in reason and will, to act or not to act, to do this or that, and so to perform deliberate actions on one's own responsibility. By free will, one shapes one's own life. Human freedom is a force for growth and maturity in truth and goodness; it attains its perfection when directed toward God, our beatitude.
>
> **1732** As long as freedom has not bound itself definitively to its ultimate good which is God, there is the possibility of choosing between good and evil, and thus of growing in perfection or of failing and sinning. This freedom characterizes properly human acts. It is the basis of praise or blame, merit, or reproach.
>
> **1733** The more one does what is good, the freer one becomes. There is no true freedom except in the service of what is good and just. The choice to disobey and do evil is an abuse of freedom and leads to "the slavery of sin" (Rom 6:17)
>
> **1734** Freedom makes man responsible for his acts to the extent that they are voluntary. Progress in virtue, knowledge of the good, and ascesis enhance the mastery of the will over its acts.

Freedom is determined to be the ability to draw one closer to God ultimately; action in opposition to that goal is slavery to disordered emotions. While Christian denominations have some variation in how they describe freedom, there is an agreement that the Holy Spirit's influence is critical in making free choices. Freedom is a gift that God gave humans when they were made in the "image of God." They were given mastery over their actions within specified limits. God also gave humans a natural desire to know and understand God. The various selections from ancient societies, the Bible, and theologians and philosophers attest to this keen interest. Thomas Aquinas, who has been cited earlier, is one of the most profound authorities on the concept of human freedom. In the encyclical *Studiorum Ducem*, Pope Pius IX writes, "the practice of the virtues disposes to the contemplation of truth, and the profound consideration of truth, in turn, gives luster and perfection to the virtues."[10]

Aquinas has a question that appears to be relevant to all people; what constitutes happiness? This subject is the first general question of morality that establishes the ultimate purpose of life. How one finds happiness dominates how we act and what we come to put into our faith? For Aqui-

---

[10] Steven J. Jensen, Living *the Good Life: A Beginner's Thomistic Ethics*, (Washington, D.C., DC: Catholic University of America Press, 2013), 78.

nas, happiness does not come from material gain, glory, or anything that we create. Happiness, or what many call joy, is a "loving vision of God."[11] Actual happiness for a believer results from a continuous unification with Christ. In John's Gospel, Jesus said, No *one can come to me unless the Father who sent me draws him, and I will raise him on the last day* (Jn 6:44). How we reach a state of fulfillment is through how we engage the various virtues God has given us. This work will not be able to describe what Aquinas did in his voluminous works comprehensively. I would direct readers to Steven J. Jensen's book, *Living the Good Life, A Beginner's Thomistic Ethics*, or G. K. Chesterton's, *St. Thomas Aquinas: The Dumb Ox* if you wish to learn more about Aquinas. Of course, if you want to become an expert in Thomistic thinking, you can also tackle his *Summa Theologica* or *Summa Contra Gentiles*, which are both multivolume works.

The second part of morality is the analysis of our voluntary actions. These voluntary actions that incline a person to act well come to perfection through the Holy Spirit's gifts (1 Cor 12:7-11), the Beatitudes (Mt 5:3-11; Lk 6:20-26), and the fruits of the Spirit (Gal 5:22-23). These actions are

---

[11] Pope Pius XI, "Library: Studiorum Ducem (On St. Thomas Aquinas)," *Catholic Culture*, accessed February 24, 2021, https://www.catholicculture.org/culture/library/view.cfm?recnum=4957, §2.

called virtues. Virtues are habits that are guided by reason. Voluntary actions are further divided into intellectual and moral virtues. Fr. John Hardon defines these two types of virtues:

> Human excellence thus defined shows itself in two forms: the habitual subordination of the senses and lower tendencies to rational rule and principle, and in the exercise of reason in the search for the contemplation of truth. The former kind of excellence is described as moral, the latter is intellectual virtue.[12]

Intellectual virtues develop worthy characteristics of the mind. Moral virtues develop the upright characteristics of the person. Jensen explains, "Intellectual helps us think well; moral virtues help us to desire well."[13]

Various mental activities that include acquired skills and knowledge are denoted as intellectual virtues because they refer to a strength for which one is inclined. Intellectual virtues come in two varieties: speculative and practical.[14]

---

[12] John A. Hardon, S.J., "Meaning of Virtue in Thomas Aquinas." *EWTN Global Catholic Television Network.* Accessed July 18, 2020. https://www.ewtn.com/catholicism/library/meaning-of-virtue-in-thomas-aquinas-12609.

[13] Ibid.

[14] Jensen, 139.

Jensen explains, "speculative virtues strengthen our understanding of truth as truth; practical virtues strengthen our application of truth to activity."[15] Speculative knowledge is notional, as in an idea of information about a particular topic. Practical knowledge is manifest in concrete achievement; something is completed, an observable event has taken place. Aquinas subdivides speculative virtues into understanding, science, and wisdom.[16] Understanding provides us with an underlying sense of principles, and science allows us to comprehend the principles' conclusions. Wisdom provides us with an overarching picture. Wisdom gives us the ability to take the individual parts and combine them into an integrated whole.

Seven principal virtues constitute the second part of morality. The first set of virtues are theological virtues. The *Catechism of the Catholic Church*, in Part Three, Article 7, teaches that "a virtue is a habitual and firm disposition to do good" (*CCC* 1803). It allows a virtuous person not merely to do kind acts but also to be the best person one can be. The *Catechism* explains, "the theological virtues are related directly to God" (*CCC* 1812). It goes on to say, "the theological virtues are the foundation of Christian moral activity; they animate it and give it its special character" (*CCC* 1813). They are evidence of the existence and action of the

---

[15] Ibid.

[16] Ibid,140.

Holy Spirit within human life. The theological virtues are considered to be gifts from God given to us gratuitously and not through any effort on our part. We are free, but not required, to accept and use them. They consist of the divine or theological virtues of faith, hope, and charity. Each of these virtues has a corresponding gift of either the Holy Spirit, a precept of the Ten Commandments that concerns it, and other virtues that may be associated. With faith, there is the gift of intelligence and knowledge. Faith is not contrary to reason or intellect but is the natural result of an understanding that is influenced by the revealed truth given to us by God. Hope contains the gift of fear, the loss of our relationship with God. We hope to have an everlasting union with God. Finally, charity is love that comes from God through our encounter with Christ and has the gift of wisdom. Charity is considered the greatest of the theological virtues. Charity is a free action, but because charity is a gift from God, we cannot obtain it through our actions. God must first give it to us as a gift before we can exercise it.

The four cardinal (aka moral) virtues comprise the second set of principles that constitute the human ability to govern our actions, direct our passions, and guide our conduct in a manner that leads to morally right acts. They are called "cardinal" because they are "hinge" (Latin: *cardo*) virtues upon which all other human qualities are based. Unlike the theological virtues that are infused knowledge given through the Holy Spirit's power, the cardinal virtues are part of the natural law. They can be refined through self-discipline and hard work.

They are the virtues that are knowable through reason and support the structure of moral life. The cardinal virtues are prudence, justice, temperance, and fortitude. Prudence directs our actions and is the essential cardinal virtue. Fortitude and Temperance concern taming our irascibility, passions, and appetites. Aquinas defines irascible passions as "those passions which regard good or bad as arduous, being difficult to obtain or avoid."[17] They belong to the irascible faculty, such as daring, fear, hope, and the like. Fortitude "is the moral virtue that ensures firmness in difficulties and constancy in the pursuit of good" (*CCC* 1808). Temperance "ensures the will's mastery over instincts and keeps desires within what is honorable" (*CCC* 1809). Justice consists of the desire to give others their just due. It is the virtue that pursues fair play. Justice takes three forms: commutative justice is based on the quid pro quo principle, Latin for "this for that." Aquinas explains commutative justice as "something that is paid to an individual on account of something of his that has been received" (ST-II, II, q.61, 2, ad).[18] It calls for a fair exchange for goods or services.

---

[17] Ibid, 139-140.

[18] Thomas Aquinas, "Whether the Passions of the Concupiscible Part Are Different from Those of the Irascible Part?" *Bible*

Distributive justice involves the relationship between one and many, as, for instance, between an individual and a group or a person and the government. In distributive justice, one is compensated based on one's merit. Distributive justice is, therefore, not an equal sharing of goods. Social justice is reflected in the relationships between individuals and groups, between one another and everyone. The common good and equal treatment are the cornerstones of social justice.

The seven virtues are the foundation of our ability to experience happiness despite the challenge of sin, anguish, and death. The virtues provide us the bridge that connects morality with our desire for happiness. Humans can access an incomplete form of happiness through the faculty of reason. From this position, we can achieve happiness in this life in proportion to the level of truth accessible to reason. Aquinas explains this as:

> So, if the ultimate felicity of man does not consist in external things which are called the goods of fortune, nor in the goods of the body, nor in the goods of the soul according to its sensitive part, nor as regards the intellective part according to the activity of the moral virtues, nor according to the intellectual virtues that are

---

Hub, accessed February 24, 2021, https://biblehub.com/library/aquinas/summa_theologica/whether_the_passions_of_the.htm.

concerned with action, that is, art and prudence—we are left with the conclusion that the ultimate felicity of man lies in the contemplation of truth.[19]

Aquinas allows that we cannot reach the perfect happiness, which he calls the *beatific vision*, here on earth. We can come to experience an imperfect state of happiness. Although there is a distinction between the two types of happiness, Aquinas' view opens up the idea that Augustine's concept of original sin does not entirely corrupt humans. Through the cardinal and theological virtues, it is possible to begin healing in this lifetime. By using the virtues of prudence, fortitude, temperance, and justice, we are given the ability to start a process of seeking God.

Moreover, in his grace, God has revealed the three additional virtues: faith, love, and hope. While true happiness is found in the knowledge of God, we can, by use of the cardinal and theological virtues, put ourselves "on the road" to that ultimate desire. Jensen sums up Aquinas' thinking as "No created good can ever fulfill our needs. Only the uncreated God, who is complete and perfect goodness, can bring us happiness."[20]

---

[19] Jensen, 105.

[20] Thomas Aquinas, "St. Thomas Aquinas – Summa Contra Gentiles - Book III (Q. 1-83)," *Genius* (Genius Media Group), accessed February 24, 2021, https://genius.com/St-thomas-

It is essential to see happiness as a commitment to living a life directed toward knowledge of God. Too often, we are willing to substitute short-term enjoyment because it satisfies the worldly desires we hold in high regard: wealth, status, prestige, etc. Happiness concerns obtaining our absolute perfection, which, by definition, can only be found in the Supreme Being, which is God.

One other thought before I move on to giving examples of both historical and ordinary everyday people who represent those who endeavor to live a virtuous life. Aquinas believed that perfect happiness is only possible in the afterlife. Buddhists and Hindus would argue that they think perfection is attainable by pointing to the Buddha, who has obtained absolute enlightenment. There is a mystical side to monotheistic religions like Christianity, Islam, and Judaism with persons like the Christian mystics, Mohammed, and many of the prophets throughout history who seem to have reached a deeper relationship with God. Aquinas' own mystical experience at the end of his life might be just such an example: perhaps he achieved a beatific vision of God, an image so sharp that it rendered all of his words obsolete. However, there can be no question: living a virtuous life places you in proximity to God, making happiness a realistic result.

---

aquinas-summa-contra-gentiles-book-iii-q-1-83-annotated,   37, §1.

Examples of Virtuous People

This section of the chapter on virtuous living will focus on some examples of holy people from the Bible and every-day people that I have encountered in my life who are dedicated to living in a way that will bring them closer to God. Three figures chosen as the archetype of virtue from the Bible are Elijah, Mary, and John the Baptist. Each of these three biblical figures embodies the life of virtue. Elijah represents the theological virtue of faith, Mary demonstrates love, and John the Baptist exemplifies hope. Of course, each of these three exhibited many more qualities of virtuous living. My goal is to illustrate how these three serve as models for anyone who wishes to live well, that is, live a life centered on reaching happiness as has been so far defined. I would then like to bring the discussion back to how every-day people whom I have known exemplify how one can live well. These people represent all of us who have suffered and sinned yet have maintained a desire to reach a higher level of awareness of how God directs lives toward good.

Elijah's popular image, a larger-than-life figure, is that of a courageous wonder-worker who calls down fire from heaven and ascends to heaven in a fiery chariot. While that makes for an exciting tale, the fact is Elijah was a deeply conflicted man, torn between a passionate idealism and a profound disappointment over his failure to achieve his ideals. Despite his profound sense of failure, Elijah's strug-

gle against King Ahab's corrupt regime and his queen, Jezebel, managed to save monotheism from being overtaken by
polytheism and, in so doing, alter the course of human history. His is an example of the struggle between the ideals of
human dignity and justice and the alternative of conven-
ience in pursuing power. This conflict permeates human
life to this very day.

Elijah's story is told in 1 Kings 17 -19 and 2 Kings 1- 2.
The story begins with Elijah proclaiming a drought is about
to occur in Israel and how God directs Elijah to go to the
widow in Zarephath. The LORD protects the widow and her
son from the famine and still more miraculously allows Elijah to resuscitate the widow's son after he had fallen ill. All
this is done because Elijah is obedient and has confidence
in how the LORD has directed him. His faith and complete
obedience to God's commands revealed to the widow that
he was a *man of God* (1 Kgs 17:24). This attitude of compliance will be the benchmark against which future obedience
will be evaluated. By his proclaiming the word of God in his
prayer for the son, he becomes not only a herald but an intercessor; Elijah is transformed into being a prophet. He is
now not only a proclaimer of the word, but he also becomes
a spokesperson for God to mediate between God and humanity.

Next, Elijah demonstrates God's power over Baal, a ge-
neric term for a pantheon of gods in the ancient Middle
East. The God of Elijah was elevated above state-supported

idolatry. Elijah can defeat the prophets of Baal, demonstrating that the LORD *God of Abraham, Isaac, and Israel, let it be known this day that you are God in Israel and that I am your servant and have done these things at your command* (1 Kgs 18:36). In this proclamation, we can see God being raised above merely being a controller of nature to intimately participating in humankind's destiny. Elijah stands between monotheism and Baal's return, championed by the Jezebel in Israel's royal court.

The next part of the story shows that Elijah has not moved the people despite his triumph. The stark realization breaks Elijah's euphoria because neither King Ahab nor the people have returned to the one God. Elijah has dropped into hopelessness. Moreover, Jezebel threatens Elijah's life, causing him to again flee for his life in the shelter of a cave. In his despair, he prays for death to come to him. Rather than go back to Israel, Elijah escapes going south to Mt. Horeb. The LORD comes to him, questioning why he fled. Elijah defends himself as being *most zealous for the LORD, the God of hosts, but the Israelites have forsaken your covenant* (1 Kgs 19:10). He is, in a sense, preparing to submit his resignation to God. At this point, Elijah is wholly centered upon his predicament. God then tells Elijah, *Go out and stand on the mountain before the LORD* (1 Kgs 19:11). He is, in a sense, calling Elijah out. God then reveals himself not through nature's power but *a light silent sound* (1 Kgs 19:12). Elijah had thought through the dramatic event of overcoming Baal's prophets the people would repent and return to God. God reveals himself to Elijah, showing that it is not the miracle that converts but through the silence's soft message. Like other flawed humans, Elijah realizes that he is looking for a big act to change people. God shows Elijah that God is not in nature's forces but is a spiritual presence inhabiting the silence. It is the silence that allows Elijah to hear the Word of God.

God repeats the question, *Why are you here, Elijah?* (1 Kgs 19:9) and commands Elijah to fulfill his call as a prophet. Elijah has matured from a religious loyalist who is an obedient servant of God to a prophet who first acts as a messenger and then mediator for humanity. He has learned to have faith that God can provide, no matter how dire the circumstances. Elijah comes to understand he must subordinate himself to the will of God. Finally, he comes to see how difficult it is for flawed humans to change their ways; change is an evolving process that takes time. The big act does not accomplish it. Instead, it is a continuous effort to live a virtuous life that will result in humanity's transformation. Elijah is an example of how God uses indistinct people to execute his plan. It is Elijah's faith that comes; as a result, God's revealing the truth to him is what allows this imperfect human to undertake God's mission to redeem the people of God.

Mary is, likewise, an ordinary person chosen by God to be Jesus' mother. Jesus is no ordinary person but the one who will aid humanity in conquering sin and its resultant separation from God. This action is accomplished through repentance, forgiveness, obedience, and following Jesus' teachings and model. Mary's concept as the "Mother of God" (*Theotokos*) is contested in the early church. By the time of the Council of Chalcedon, 451 CE, the term's use becomes an accepted part of the dogma. Mary's role in salvation history is contrasted with Eve's in Genesis. Genesis shows the connection between the first woman, Eve, who is represented as a "mediatrix" tasked with lifting humanity to God. Instead, she becomes the antimediatrix by encouraging Adam to listen to the serpent (devil). Mary is the new Eve, from whom the new Adam emerges. In other parts of the Old Testament, Mary is compared with four women: Rebecca, Rachel, Judith, and Esther. Rebecca is the progenitor of the twelve tribes of Israel; Rachel is the mother of Joseph who saves his people from famine; Judith defeats the enemy by cutting off its head, and Esther, as Queen, tends to her people. Mary fulfills each of these roles. She is seen as the Ark of the New Covenant through the annunciation; Mary has become the special dwelling place of God's glory.

The story of Bathsheba in 2 Samuel 11:2-4 is familiar to many and would not, upon first glance, appear to be a "type" of Mary. As her story develops, we come to see her as a wise counselor to Solomon. She intercedes on the part of Adonias, fourth son of David by Haggith, deprived of the throne, and best known for his failed attempts to usurp Is-

rael's throne after David's death (1 Kgs 1:5-8). It was directly after this treachery that Bathsheba goes to Solomon to
speak on behalf of Adonias. Bathsheba, the Queen Mother,
has extraordinary influence as she sits at the king's right
hand. The people know that they can go to her with their
petitions, and the king will listen to her. Bathsheba's role is
the most complete of the women in the Old Testament as
she is in the line from which the Savior will be born. Bathsheba is the Queen Mother of Israel during its most successful period; Mary is the Mother and Queen of all people.
As the *Memorare* (a prayer for the help of Mary) says,
"Never was it known that anyone who fled to thy protection, implored thy help or sought intercession was left un-
aided."

The woman in Proverbs 31 is the model for Christian
women. The Church identifies in the valiant woman "characteristics of the Mother of God, whom Christians since
ancient times have invoked as the Seat of Wisdom."[21]
Bergsma and Pitre identify three specific verses in Proverbs
31 that point to the valiant woman being Mary. *She opens
her mouth with wisdom, and the teaching of kindness is on
her tongue (31:26). Her children arise and call her blessed"
(31:28), and "Many women have done excellently, but you
surpass them all (31:29).* The authors acknowledge these
thoughts in the New Testament in Luke 1:38-42 and John

---

[21] Jensen, 194.

2:5.[22] St. Paul mentions Mary (although he does not give her name) only once in Galatians 4:4-5 and this by reference as he writes: *But when the fullness of the time came, God sent forth his Son, born of a woman, born under the Law, so that he might redeem those who were under the Law, that we might receive the adoption as sons.*

Mary is the one who assures the genuineness of the Incarnation in its human element. Paul, explaining that Jesus was born of a woman without a human father, lays the foundation for proposing a virginal conception and divine nature of the birth event. Paul's message in Galatians 4:4-5 is Jesus' presence is the *result of a divine act of sending* (Gal 4:4) and *that he came to redeem those who were under the law* (Gal 4:5).

It is through Luke that we most clearly see Mary's obedience and love being confirmed. Luke gives us several pericopes in which Mary's role supports the divinity of Jesus. First, in the Annunciation, the use of the phrase *the LORD is with you* (Lk 1:28) is an announcement that a formidable task is now before Mary. The message is the fulfillment of the hope of a Messiah is near. As *Son of the Most High* (Lk 1:32), Luke presents the idea of Jesus' divinity. For Mary, this assigns a divine aspect as "the Mother of God." Mary accepts her role by her devoted reply, *Let it happen to me as you say* (Lk 1:38). Mary showed her love for Jesus, not

---

[22] Bergsma and Pitre, 617.

simply through the obedient response to God. She manifests love in her nurturing, teaching, and following of Jesus even to the Cross. Elizabeth Johnson uses the example of the *Magnificat* as a prophetic song giving an image of Mary that reveals her as a poor woman for whom God, despite her low status, has done great things.[23] She is the model of those God chooses to favor, a first-century Galilean peasant woman. In the second part of the *Magnificat*, Luke uses the biblical theme of reversal to demonstrate the marginalized while the arrogant are losers. *He has thrown down the rulers from their throne but lifted up the lowly* (Lk 1:52). Johnson writes that Mary is singing a liberating song in which "Luke depicts her as the spokeswoman for God's redemptive justice."[24] Mary's love for humanity is established in later writing within the Church observing Mary's role as an intercessor for those who come to her for assistance. Through her strong bond of love with Christ, it is believed that she can act on behalf of others. Because of God's gift of being the Mother of God, Mary can share that love with others. Mary

---

[23] Ibid.

[24] Elizabeth A. Johnson, "Mary, Mary, Quite Contrary," *U.S. Catholic* 68, no. 12 (December 2003): pp. 12-17, http://search. ebscohost.com.ezp.slu.edu/login.aspx?direct=true&db=f5h&AN =11487970&site=eds-live, 14.

becomes the first disciple through her Son's love and the model for all Christians regarding her giving nature.

The third biblical character to be discussed is John the Baptist. Matthew 11:2-7 gives us an account concerning John, which can be read as a story of questioning his initial reaction to Jesus expressed in Matthew 3:13-15: *Then Jesus came from Galilee to John at the Jordan to be baptized by him. John tried to prevent him, saying, "I need to be baptized by you, and yet you are coming to me? In reply, Jesus said to him, 'Allow it now, for thus, it is fitting for us to fulfill all righteousness.' Then he allowed him.* It appears in those passages that John sees Jesus as the hoped-for Messiah. The rest of the pericope shows the Spirit of God descending upon Jesus and declaring him to be *"my beloved Son"* (Mt 3:17). Another interpretation suggested by Reginald Fuller in his commentary on this reading for the Third Sunday of Advent in the A Cycle is the real question, *"Can we believe that he is the Coming One, or must we look for another?"*[25] Jesus' response in Matthew 11:5-6 is taken from Isaiah, where the prophet presents God's plan in the positive aspects of ending pride, ignorance, and injustice (Is 29:17-24; 35:5-10; 61). John's question for which he sends his disciples is not for his enlightenment; he has already accepted that Jesus is the answer to his hope for a Messiah. John already knows that Jesus is the way to an everlasting relation-

---

[25] Ibid, 15-16.

ship with God. John is the sign that one has been sent ahead to prepare the way. He is announcing the kingdom is imminent and that Jesus is the way to salvation. Fuller says, "John stands at the threshold of the new age. He is the last of the prophets and, like them, still points forward to the kingdom of heaven and the coming of the Messiah."[26]

The common denominator about these three individuals is they either came from or chose to live a low-status and often lonely life. Each of them had suffered personally yet ultimately were authentic in their love for God and desired ultimate happiness. Mary, the Mother of God, and John the Baptist had the advantage of knowing Jesus Christ to realize God's promise. Elijah, the prophet, had his faith, despite the setback he experiences. Each experienced miracles yet came to understand that proof of God's saving grace did not come through the mighty acts of nature but in the silence that allowed the hearing of God's Word. When we look at these three people's lives, they are extraordinary in their ability to see God through the trials and tribulations of their life. In John's case, it meant his death at the hands of a despot. Elijah barely escaped execution by a pagan Queen, and Mary had to endure seeing her beloved Son die, in apparent disgrace, on the Cross.

---

[26] Reginald H. Fuller and Daniel Westberg. *Preaching the Lectionary: The Word of God for the Church Today,* (Revised Edition), (Collegeville, MN: Liturgical Press, 1984), 7-10.

I would agree that almost none of us will ever be in the dire position of Elijah, Mary, and John the Baptist. Christ's sacrifice has provided the path to salvation. Thomas Rausch explains how Jesus shows the way to salvation. He first points out that despite apparent failure, remained confident that God would vindicate him."[27] His mission was not a failure. He says that Jesus refused to meet evil with evil allows God to reveal the life-giving power of love, overcoming death. God's supremacy is revealed in Jesus' ability to overcome the disgrace of death on a cross through his resurrection. Jesus is the source of our salvation, as, through Christ and his Spirit, we can be intimately related to God. Rausch says, "The stories of people whose lives were radically changed by their encounter with Jesus … means God is there."[28] The good news for each of us is that through Christ, we can come to know God. Yet, such a journey is not easy and requires living within the virtues that have been discussed herein.

Within my life, I have had the opportunity to be in the presence of many people who have maintained a strong faith in Jesus Christ while overcoming adversity. Their experience, which I will briefly describe, validates that living a

---

[27] Ibid.

[28] Thomas P. Rausch, *Who Is Jesus? An Introduction to Christology*, (Collegeville, MN: Liturgical Press, 2003), 110.

virtuous life, while not alleviating all misery, does allow one to continue the journey of happiness.

I am fortunate to have a group of friends for whom faith life is central to who they are and how they act. It is a group of men and women as young as their mid-twenties with growing families and all the stress of earning a living, keeping up with children's activities, and in some cases, furthering their education. The group also includes middle-aged and retired people, many of whom are now "empty nesters." We have come to know each other through Church activities such as That Man Is You," Parish Renewal meetings, Christ Renews His Parish, and Acts retreats. Many of us have also participated in retreats conducted by Jesuits at the White House Retreat Center in St. Louis, Trappists at the Abbey of Gethsemane in Trappist, Kentucky, Benedictines at Subiaco Abby in Subiaco, Arkansas, and the Casa Maria Retreat House sponsored by the Sister Servants of the Eternal Word near Birmingham, Alabama. Several of us have met on Saturday mornings to discuss the reading for Mass for over 30 years. There is the active support of the Parish, the Archdiocesan Annual Appeal, and Catholic Charities organizations. This group of people also serves as Eucharistic Ministers, both in Church and for those who cannot attend Mass. They are lectors and ushers, and they are actively involved in both the catechesis of the youth and adult education and the Rite of Christian Initiation (RCIA). I offer this resume because one could easily believe this group is immune to suffering due to their fidelity. One might posit that their faithfulness has earned them protection from suffering. Yet, this characterization is completely inaccurate.

Within the group, there have been times of great pain. Miscarriages of babies have occurred with several couples, as well as adult children's death and employment loss for long periods. Several have borne acute and chronic illnesses, including cancer, congestive heart failure, diabetes, and chronic arthritis. There have been instances of children divorcing and leaving the Church, following post-modern distrust of anything related to religion. Saying this is a protected class of people due to their faith suggests a superstitious understanding of God's action in the world.

They share the desire to have an intimate and enduring relationship of love with Jesus and their fellow beings. They desire to invite others to share in Christ's love. They do not have a transactional connection to Christ. That is, it is not an if/then proposition. In its place, they have unconditional faith in God's love and mercy, enduring hope that the promise of Christ's life, death, and resurrection is present within their lives. They know that they can participate in the kingdom now and hereafter due to God's grace. They are glad to share that love with others. Their faith is not contingent upon outward signs. Instead, they have a relationship that embraces Christ's ideal of love and the courage to live a life directed at the happiness of knowing God.

The focus is not on the immediate gain but everlasting life. As one friend stated, "It is my goal to get to heaven and invite all others to join me." Each of these people is intentional in their effort to have their will, informed by reason, to direct their actions.

As I noted earlier, they are people who seek to live a life Pinckaers' terms "Freedom for Excellence." That means that they seek to act in ways that seek truth and happiness beyond momentary pleasure. We often settle for personal comfort, accumulate material goods, and meet our desires as a definition of happiness. The problem is that happiness defined as a fleeting instance of utilitarianism, or hedonism, promotes actions that maximize physical pleasure or well-being for the affected individuals. Pinckaers defines the difference between pleasure and enduring happiness (joy) this way: Pleasure is an agreeable sensation, a passion caused by contact with some *exterior* good. Joy, however is something *interior;* joy is the direct effect of an *excellent action.*[29]

Happiness is attained by developing good habits established progressively with education, involvement with others, directed toward good, and internalized; they become your virtues. That is, actions are manifestations of who one is internally and are done in humility. Actions are not self-serving but are meant to use the gifts given to serve a larger whole. It comes from the freedom I talked about earlier that

---

[29] Pinckaers, 78.

is a result of living a virtuous life. Happiness is, thus, not only those things that lead to an impression of material success. It includes the learning and experience we gain in suffering, which is accepted with courage. Understanding is what we come to experience in life as an opportunity to become imitators of Christ and come to know and love God even more completely.

Summary

The chapter deals with specific thoughts and examples concerning how one can live life in such a way as to prepare for the kingdom. It also provides some examples of extraordinary and ordinary people who have lived remarkably virtuous lives. Seven principal virtues constitute the second part of morality. The first set of virtues are theological virtues. *The Catechism of the Catholic Church*, in Part Three, Article 7, teaches that "a virtue is a habitual and firm disposition to do good" (*CCC* 1803). It allows a virtuous person not merely to do kind acts but also to be the best person one can be. The four cardinal (aka moral) and three theological virtues comprise the second set of principles that constitute the human ability to govern our actions, direct our passions, and guide our conduct in a manner that leads to morally right acts. The seven virtues are the foundation of our ability to experience happiness despite the challenge of sin, anguish, and death. The virtues provide us the bridge that connects morality with our desire for happiness.

Suggested Reading

Morality, The Catholic View by Servais Pinckaers, O.P., has an exceptionally clear description of "happiness" and how one can find true freedom through the pursuit of happiness.

Living the Good Life: A Beginner's Thomistic Ethics by Steven Jensen deals primarily with Aquinas's philosophy with particular attention to his teaching's practicality to our world today.

St. Thomas Aquinas: The Dumb Ox by C.K. Chesterton has often been called the best summary of who Thomas Aquinas was and what he taught that continues to impact us even today. It is a must reading for those interested in Thomas Aquinas, the person.

A Shorter Summa: The Essential Philosophical Passages of St. Thomas Aquinas' Summa Theologica, edited and explained by Peter Kreeft, is a great way to "dangle your feet in the water" if you are not ready to tackle Aquinas's multi-volume *Summa Theologica*. The book contains many of the most influential sections of Aquinas' work with the editor's helpful footnotes.

Thomas Aquinas in 50 Pages by Taylor R. Marshall is a short primer on the theology and philosophy of Thomas Aquinas.

Mere Christianity, written by C. S. Lewis, expands his radio talks given on BBC Radio during World War II. In the book, the author makes a case for the existence of God. He then proceeds to outline what, for him, are the fundamental principles of Christianity. In *Book III: Christian Behavior*, the work provides an excellent definition of the cardinal (Chapter 2) and theological virtues (Chapters 9-12).

Chapter Seven

Informed Consent, What Does It Really Mean?

For you were called for freedom, brothers.
But do not use this freedom as
an opportunity for the flesh;
rather serve one another through love. (John 5:13)

In previous chapters, I have discussed freedom and virtuous living. Both of these concepts are components of the discussion concerning informed consent. Freedom is contained within the will, a component of the human soul. The will contains the power of self-determination, which is a deliberate choice to act that derives from our ability to reason: it is thus commonly designated the rational appetite. The will is more forceful than the lower appetites (physical and emotional desires). It exercises a preferential control; its specific act, therefore, when it is in full exercise, consists of selecting by the light of reason. Its object is the good in general; its responsibility is choosing among different forms of good.

Freedom, then, is the inclination to pursue what is right and suitable and avoid what is evil. The cardinal virtues come into play in that they perfect the elements of the human soul. Justice perfects the will; prudence, the intellect; courage, the irascible appetite (hope and despair; courage, fear, and anger); and temperance, the concupiscible appetite (love and hatred, desire and aversion, joy, and sadness). Our intentional action, which desires to have a life described as "well-lived" that we find employing the cardinal virtues, provides the path to flourishing and freedom. Virtuous living, therefore, includes the ability to make informed decisions about personal relationships, spiritual desires, ethical decisions, and self-determination with regard to health care needs.

This chapter will focus on the central importance of informed consent, allowing one to make reasoned decisions for those with a life-limiting illness. Note I did not say end–of-life, although that is undoubtedly a factor to be addressed. Informed consent is directed at allowing the individual to flourish within the opportunities available to him or her. The conversation will also delve into family and friends' roles in supporting and enhancing the community of love in which each of us lives. The chapter will also provide a foundation for Primary Care Providers (physicians, physicians assistants, advanced practice nurses) to prepare to have what Angelo Volandes calls "*The Conversation.*"

Let's begin the discussion by discussing how informed consent is treated within the medical community as a *pro forma* exercise. There is often virtually no discussion between the person to be cared for and the provider of care.

Frequently, this is due to time constraints or the patient's reluctance to discuss what they believe will be an unpleasant and frightening conversation. I know of individuals who have family histories of a chronic, congenital condition who prefer not to discuss the subject. This approach suggests the person might believe talking about something will make it happen. It is more likely they believe nothing can be done, so "why talk about it." An American Medical Association website (https://www.ama-assn.org/delivering-care/ethics/ informed-consent) describes informed consent with the following definition:

Informed consent to medical treatment is fundamental in both ethics and law. Patients have the right to receive information and ask questions about recommended treatments so that they can make well-considered decisions about care. Successful communication in the patient-physician relationship fosters trust and supports shared decision-making. The process of informed consent occurs when communication between a patient and physician results in the patient's authorization or agreement to undergo a specific medical intervention. In seeking a patient's informed consent (or the consent of the patient's surrogate if the patient lacks decision-making capacity or declines to participate in making decisions), physicians should:

(a) Assess the patient's ability to understand relevant medical information and the implications of treatment alternatives and to make an independent, voluntary decision.

(b) Present relevant information accurately and sensitively, in keeping with the patient's preferences for receiving medical information. The physician should include information about:

1. The diagnosis (when known)
2. The nature and purpose of recommended interventions
3. The burdens, risks, and expected benefits of all options, including forgoing treatment

(c) Document the informed consent conversation and the patient's (or surrogate's) decision in the medical record in some manner. When the patient/surrogate has provided specific written consent, the consent form should be included in the record.

When a decision must be made urgently in emergencies, the patient cannot participate in decision-making, and the patient's surrogate is not available, a physician may initiate treatment without prior informed consent. In such situations, the physician should inform the patient/surrogate at the earliest opportunity and obtain consent for ongoing treatment in keeping with these guidelines. (*AMA Principles of Medical Ethics: I, II, V, VIII*)

In most interactions with caregivers, I would submit that there is the desire to be assured that the patient is as fully informed as the AMA guidelines recommend. Yet, the time required to explain procedures and the patient's health literacy level can limit the achievement of the AMA guidelines' goals. Besides, the availability of easy access to information on the internet has created a new patient self-diagnosis phenomenon. My daughter-in-law, a family practice physician, and other physicians I have talked with acknowledge the value of access to information. They also recognize the problems it presents when not combined with discussions with caregivers. Thus, when I talk about patients' health literacy, I refer to either too little or too much information to interfere with listening actively and using one's intellect and reasoning ability to come to prudent decisions.

Throughout this section of the book, I will look at each component of this definition. I will avoid giving general commentary on how well each element is executed except where I have firsthand observation or strong empirical evidence. My purpose in the examination is to outline how this process can support the effort to increase the person's opportunity to flourish. Human flourishing used in the way I am describing it is an effort to achieve fulfillment within the context of a broader community of individuals. It is a community that accepts the human person's dignity and respects the common good for all. The goal of life proposed in this book is one of achieving happiness. To reach that level, I have argued that living a virtuous life built around the cardinal and theological virtues is essential. The dignity of the human person, realized in community with others, is the standard against which all parts of life must be measured.

One critical component that enables a human to thrive is the ability to make well-considered decisions concerning their health and welfare. Prudence allows one to discern an appropriate course of action. Courage gives one the ability to confront their fears. These two cardinal virtues are central to the process of informed consent. For these virtues to be useful requires one more critical component: competence. For a person to process the information that allows an individual to make a well-considered choice necessitates a certain level of capacity. Capacity does not refer to any test of intelligence. Capacity is determined by meeting specific criteria that include:

- Understanding what the medical treatment is, its purpose and nature, and why it is being proposed. This information should be conveyed using as little technical jargon as possible.

- Being aware of the benefits, risks, and alternative options available.
- The recognition of the potential consequences of not receiving the proposed treatment.
- An awareness of the financial responsibility that will accrue to the individual.
- Allowance of patients to consult with other professionals (including seeking spiritual guidance), family, and friends concerning the course of action to be chosen ultimately.
- The ability of the individual to retain the information and weigh the pros and cons to decide.
- The demonstrated ability of the individual to articulate the decision to others.

In other words, competence is a requirement for a person to exercise autonomy. Competence includes being able to obtain the information required to make an informed decision. Information gathering can consist of a consultation with other professionals and spiritual advisors trained in bioethics. What I propose expands on the elements outlined in the AMA guidelines because the choices one makes, especially regarding care to be received in the event of a life-limiting illness, impact the individual and those others of significance in his or her life.

Typically, patients or their advocates, if they are unable or considered not competent to speak for themselves, should sign an informed consent form. The caregiver should also document the conversation and conclusions in the patient's medical record. Often, the Informed Consent process is not managed by the caregiver. Instead, it becomes an administrative process completed at the time of admission to the hospital or before an office visit or procedure. It is not altogether clear whether the patient or the family have the opportunity to fully comply with the entirety of the process of informed consent. The result is that we often meet the process's administrative and legal requirements but not the intent to assure that the patient has both the capacity to understand what is being offered or the opportunity to explore other options. The patient and family in this case are not making an informed decision in the fullest sense of the concept. While this may be acceptable (although I disagree with that position) for persons without a diagnosis of a life-limiting illness, it is not for the person who is now facing his or her mortality. It is no longer a notional concept but has become real. Because assuring informed consent is obtained, not just an administrative or legal obligation as necessitated, the development of an Advance Care Plan, which is designed to be adjusted based upon the patient's progression in the illness process, is preferable.

Advance Care Plans, also known as living wills or "durable power of attorney," have been given a great deal of exposure since the enactment of the Affordable Care Act (a.k.a. Obamacare) and the approval of reimbursement to physicians or other qualified professionals beginning in January 2016. The goals, as stated in the description of new measures to the 80 Fed. Reg. 39840 (July 10, 2015), are that "advance care planning ensures that the health care plan is consistent with the patient's wishes and preferences" and "increased advance care planning among the elderly is expected to result in enhanced patient autonomy and reduced hospitalizations and in-hospital deaths" (§39882). These two goals appear on the surface to be desirable to assure patients give informed consent that is consistent with their wishes. The rule also provides value to the idea of advance care planning by compensating caregivers for undertaking these difficult discussions. The downside is that it formalizes the process with requirements that stipulate what is necessary to obtain reimbursement. These rules can have the effect of moving the process back to primarily administrative duty. The concern that the rule, while having good intentions, would have unanticipated consequences that would diminish the impact on patient well-being is the very issue addressed. The Office of the General Counsel for the United States Council of Catholic Bishops outlined the concerns in a letter dated September 4. 2015, sent to the Centers for Medicare and Medicaid Services (https://www.usccb.org/sites/default/files/about/general-counsel/rulemaking/upload/Comments-Advance-Directives-Medicare-9-15.pdf).

Anthony R. Picarello, Jr., Associate General Secretary, General Counsel, and Michael Moses, Associate General Counsel, addressed several issues troubling to the U. S. Bishops. Although they acknowledged:

> The Church has a long and rich tradition on the parameters for such decision making, providing concepts and distinctions that have long played an important role in secular medical ethics as well. We hold that each human life, at every stage and in every condition, has an innate dignity and that acts or omissions directly intended to take an innocent life are never justified. We also recognize that the moral obligation to preserve one's life has limits, particularly when the means offered for life may be useless or impose burdens that are disproportionate to their benefits.[1]

the concerns expressed revolved around three issues:

1. The rules validated only those types of advance care planning that either required the designation of a

---

[1] Anthony R. Picarello, and Michael F. Moss. *United States Conference of Catholic Bishops*, September 4, 1915. http://www.usccb.org/about/general-counsel/rulemaking/upload/Comments-Advance-Directives-Medicare-9-15.pdf.

surrogate (I call it the advocate) or a formal document such as advanced directives. The rule gave no status to discussions that had been held and not documented with friends and relatives.

2. The rule appeared aimed at reducing health care costs rather than patient autonomy.

3. There was no specific reference to other government regulations that prohibited reimbursement for procedures that might be facilitate assisted suicide.

On behalf of the U.S. Bishops, the attorneys urged the final rules to incorporate the following elements in the final regulations.

1. Acknowledge the full range of advance care planning options, including those which rely on discussion and collaboration among family members instead of on pre-packaged documents that may be biased toward withdrawal of treatment;

2. Caution patients about the need to read any material carefully before signing it, to ensure that it adequately protects the individual patient's well-being and values, and inform them that additional resources may be available from their religious denomination or other sources of moral guidance;

3. Completely exclude counseling and documents that
   present lethal actions such as assisted suicide or euthanasia as treatment options;
4. Reflect the current law's commitment to an "equali-
   ty of life" standard that upholds life with a disability
   or permanent impairment as having inherent
   worth—explicitly referencing the "The Patient Self-
   Determination Act of 1990, the Assisted Suicide
   Funding Act of 1997, and Section 1302 of the Affordable Care Act.[2]

These are legitimate concerns about advance care planning that can be overcome by intentional attention to pro-
tecting each person's dignity as one who is made in God's
image. A well-known program begun by the Gundersen
Lutheran Health System Foundation in La Crosse, Wisconsin, is Respecting Choices®, initiated by Bud Hammes,
Ph.D., the system' Clinical Ethicist at that time. In 2000,
they offered the first course to train facilitators in La
Crosse, Wisconsin. La Crosse is now well known for its
success in assisting residents in having a conversation about
what they wish at the end of life. These discussions are not
"death-bed" conversations. Instead, they focus on the
things that are of value to the person while still actively engaged in the process. In a September 2014 article in *Forbes*

---

[2] Ibid.

Magazine by Craig Hatkoff, Rabbi Irvin Kula, and Zack Levine entitled "How to Die in America: Welcome To La Crosse, Wisconsin," the authors noted that advance care planning could potentially improve the "tenor of care" during the inevitable end-of-life process. They discussed the legal document referred to as a living will, durable power of attorney, or health care proxy. These are legal documents often drawn up by an attorney or templates that are created by state authorities. While they serve to identify direction to care-givers, they aim to reduce care costs as the actual goal.[3] Of course, this is an important goal when one sees the cost of care, especially at the end of life, continuing to increase at a pace that exceeds other goods and services in the economy. Our ability to maintain the heartbeat and breathing of a person, even after serious illness or injury, is almost unlimited. It has been estimated that nearly 30% of Medicare expenditures are for treatment in the last months of life.

There is no serious opposition to assuring that individuals get adequate treatment irrespective of age or health condition. There is, however, a compelling argument concerning a question I have posed to physicians on numerous

---

[3] Craig Hatkoff, Irvin Kula, and Zack Levine, "How To Die In America: Welcome To La Crosse, Wisconsin," *Forbes* (Forbes Magazine, October 4, 2014), https://forbes.com/sites/offwhite papers/2014/09/23/how-to-die-in-america-welcome-to-la-crosse /#2d005c0be8c6.

occasions: "Are we doing **_to_** or **_for_** the patient?" What good can this treatment do *for* this person? What harm can it do *to* them? This questioning in ethics is called weighing the benefits and burdens of an action. The "Ethical and Religious Directives for Catholic Health Care" states: "The task of medicine is to care even when it cannot cure." It further states,

> Reflections on the innate dignity of all human life in all its dimensions and on the purpose of medical care is indispensable for formulating a true moral judgment about the use of technology to maintain life.[4]

The authors of the *Forbes* article suggest that the critical question to evaluate is whether we address what the Institute of Medicine 2014 report entitled "Dying in America: Improving Quality and Honoring Preferences Near the End of Life" states as the real goal? The report concludes that we should be focused on "a person-centered, family-oriented approach that honors individual preferences and promotes quality of life through the end of life should be a national

---

[4] United States Conference of Catholic Bishops, "Part 5, Issues in Care for the Seriously Ill and Dying, Introduction," In *Ethical and Religious Directives for Catholic Health Care Services* (Washington, D.C.: United States Conference of Catholic Bishops, 2018), 28.

priority."[5] The dignity of the individual is the foremost concern of those organizations which have rigorously addressed the issue in a way that is attentive to assisting the person in flourishing. Again, this begs that we look at the cardinal and theological virtues. Prudence is required to discern the appropriate course of action with which to proceed. Courage (fortitude) allows the person to meet the fear of the unknown with hope. Justice allows that all will be treated in an equitable manner concerning their right to decision-making guided by faith in God's presence to comfort, love (charity) for humankind, and desire to have them be part of the kingdom of God. A conversation that is appealing to the dignity of the person is a far cry from Sarah Palin's "Death Panel" description of the discussion each of us is entitled to have concerning how we wish to be cared for by our health care providers.

Concern for each person's dignity is the theme that is consistent in the values statements of religiously sponsored and secular for-profit and not-for-profit health care organizations. I noted earlier that Respecting Choices* is a program that is the model for focusing on the fundamental value of dignity of the person as the center for all advance care planning. This concern for the respect of a person's ability to "have a say" concerning their wishes and desires

---

[5] Hatkoff, Kula, and Levine.

about how they will live their lives. Bud Hammes was, in his own words,

> Struck by the frequency of moral distress experienced by both families and physicians faced with critical choices about treatments for patients who lacked decision-making capacity to participate in their healthcare decisions. What appeared striking to Hammes about these instances was that the patients were typically older, they had prolonged periods of worsening health, and there was ample opportunity of engaging the patients in planning. It wasn't that patients were making the decision not to plan. Rather, there was nothing in the healthcare system that helped them to plan, and health professionals had no training or workflows to make it happen.[6]

Respecting Choices® has broadened its reach to have trained advance care planning facilitators in most states in the United States and many international locations. Respecting Choices® represents "best practices." This designation can be defined as a technique or methodology that, through experience and research, has proven to lead to the

---

[6] Hammes, Bud. "History of Respecting Choices®." *Respecting Choices.* https://respectingchoices.org/about-us/history-of-respecting-choices/.

desired result reliably. Additionally, the best practice must be one that can be replicated in various settings without prohibitive costs. My own experience with Respecting Choices® supports my understanding that not only is it a best practice, but it is also intentional in its effort to support "person-centered" care. Moreover, it is suitable for all types of health care providers, including those that abide by the US Conference of Catholic Bishops' *"Ethical and Religious Directives for Catholic Health Care Services,"* Sixth Edition, Part Five.[7] I would encourage the reader to learn more about Respecting Choices® by visiting their website: https://respectingchoices.org.

Advance care planning is a critical starting point in the process of having real informed consent. The conversation is appropriate at any age as long as one recognizes the need to update one's wishes regularly to ensure they are consistent with the current conditions of health, lifestyle, and family in which one is living. This regular updating anticipates that health and other life factors are not static, and changes will occur. The discovery of an illness that has the potential to be life-limiting is something many will face during their lifetimes. A diagnosis of a life-limiting health issue is often met with the idea that "we will fight this dreaded condition," or alternatively, "we choose to do nothing until the condition becomes unmanageable." Both

---

[7] United States Catholic Bishops, 25-28.

of these options suggest that how I live is conditioned upon external forces (e.g., a medical procedure or newly discovered cure). It is crucial to have medical technology and research benefits to assist in dealing with health issues in a time of need. Nevertheless, I would suggest a third alternative that allows you to live your life as freely as possible while pursuing the desired result. That alternative is palliative care.

Before World War II, hospital care was, of necessity, mostly supportive. Few pharmaceuticals could provide the alleviation of symptoms and even outright cures that are available today. After the war, the United States government began to direct money into the health care system primarily due to the needs of a post-war population of veterans and the "baby-boom." The development of new technologies, pharmaceuticals, and effective specific treatments for disease became the main focus of medicine. With the advances in technology and the discovery of life-extending and even life-saving medication came an increase in medical specialization.

Medical specialization is not a new phenomenon, as history records evidence of physicians specializing in specific ailments as far back as Galen (129 CE-216 CE), a Greek physician and surgeon in the Roman empire. The Association of American Medical Colleges lists 20 specialties in medicine, most with subspecialties that bring the number of specialty/subspecialties to just under 200.[8] In surgery alone, there are 31 areas of specialization. It is not hard to imagine a medically complex patient having three or more physicians attending to the various disorders the person may be experiencing.

A medically complex patient has multiple medical conditions. The medically complex patient is not just a concentration of physical conditions in one person that can be addressed individually. The medically complex patient also brings socioeconomic factors, including financial resources, family dynamics, and health literacy differences. Often, mental illnesses, such as depression, addiction, and anxiety, lead to poor compliance with caregivers' directions. The combination of physical, emotional, and socioeconomic influences can result in a patient and family having expectations that may not be easily be accommodated.

Misunderstanding and subsequent mistrust of the providers can emerge as the patient or family projects motives of discrimination, withholding of care for economic reasons, or caregiver incompetence. The medically complex patient is one in whom care coordination among providers is of utmost importance. That coordination becomes virtu-

---

[8] SGU Pulse, "The Ultimate List of Medical Specialties - Explore Options," (St. George University, December 11, 2017), https://www.sgu.edu/blog/medical/ultimate-list-of-medical-specialties/.

ally impossible in situations where the patient has no primary care provider (PCP) or Medical Home.

The Primary Care Collaborative defines a medical home as,

> The medical home is best described as a model or philosophy of primary care that is patient-centered, comprehensive, team-based, coordinated, accessible, and focused on quality and safety. It has become a widely accepted model for how primary care should be organized and delivered throughout the health care system and is a philosophy of health care delivery that encourages providers and care teams to meet patients where they are, from the most simple to the most complex conditions. Patients are treated with respect, dignity, and compassion and enables strong and trusting relationships with providers and staff. Above all, the medical home is not a final destination; instead, it is a model for achieving primary care excellence so that care is received in the right place, at the right time, and in the manner that best suits a patient's needs.[9]

This definition is the ideal for which legislative acts like the Affordable Care and Patient Affordability Act was intended. The idea was to break down barriers to access by

---

[9] Online at https://www.pcpcc.org/

providing nearly universal health insurance for all citizens. Some states have even advocated having health insurance available to all residents irrespective of citizenship status. The goal of establishing medical homes as a standard is far from realized.

Nevertheless, a model for the community-based medical home has demonstrated a great deal of success. These organizations are formed under the provisions of the Federally Qualified Health Center (FQHC). An FQHC is a designation offered by the Bureau of Primary Health Care and the Centers for Medicare and Medicaid Services of the U. S. Department of Health and Human Services, funded under the Health Center Consolidation Act (Section 330 of the Public Health Service Act). It provides enhanced Medicaid reimbursement to facilitate low-income or disabled, elderly, and dependent children. The centers provide primary care services in underserved areas. They must meet a stringent set of requirements, including providing care on a sliding fee scale based on ability to pay and operating under a governing board that includes patients. In addition to primary care, FQHCs incorporate access to obstetric/gynecological services, pediatric care, discounted pharmaceuticals, mental health, substance abuse, and oral health services in areas where economic, geographic, or cultural barriers limit access to affordable health care services. Although FQHCs are primarily designed for underserved populations, they can serve as a coordinated care model for all payor groups. Unfortunately, Americans have been reluctant to embrace concepts that revolve around coordinated care, such as Health Maintenance Organizations (HMOs).

Health consumers (that is how we are viewed) in the United States have become accustomed to a health system providing what people want when they want it. Moreover, the health care system benefits most from illness, not health. I discussed this characteristic of the American health care delivery system earlier. It is a system driven by consumer emotional desire and short-term gratification. This demand/supply feature of health care delivery contrasts with the concept of freedom for self-determination based upon each to discern. It is a freedom that seeks ways that allow humans (and all God's creations) to flourish. Michael Panicola and co-authors in *An Introduction to Health Care Ethics: Theological Foundations, Contemporary Issues, and Controversial Cases* identify discernment as "the skill or virtue of perceiving and distinguishing degrees of value between diverse factors when making decisions."[10] Discernment includes the virtue of prudence but is not exclusively a product of reason. The authors point out that discernment includes a spiritual component involving introspec-

---

[10] Michael R. Panicola, David M. Belde, John Paul Slosar, and Mark F. Repenshek, *An Introduction to Health Care Ethics: Theological Foundations, Contemporary Issues, and Controversial Cases,* (Winona, MN: Anselm Academic, 2007), 65.

tion and the contemplation of thoughts, desires, and conduct combined with the ability to reason as essential in arriving at informed decisions that allow the person to flourish. Part of that discernment process includes the ability to engage and actively listen to health care providers who are part of an integrated and health-focused system.

In Chapter 9, I will spend a great deal of time identifying the elements of a health care system that defines virtuous coordination of care. In addition to the need to have a more coordinated primary care system, I would maintain the need to be able to serve those persons who have been diagnosed with a life-limiting (note, I did not say life-ending) condition that, with proper care, can facilitate the ability of the person to flourish.

In the concluding chapter, I would like to discuss health care services aimed explicitly toward assisting persons with a life-limiting illness to flourish. To complete that subject, I want to return to the discussion of palliative care. As I noted earlier, before the middle of the 20th century, most hospital care was supportive (palliative) in nature. The treatment goal was focusing on preventing or at least relieving suffering on the part of the patient. It was the experience of wars and discovering what seemed to be miracle drugs that converted hospitals to be viewed as life-saving places. In addition, there was the emergence of health insurance provided by employers, which was expanded during World War II. In 1946, the Hill-Burton Act provided government incentive financing to construct hospitals that had fallen into disrepair due to the Depression and during WWII. Ironically, the Act was a successful effort to deflect interest in passing President Harry Truman's plan for a prepaid health insurance plan for all Americans. Universal health care insurance was discussed as early as Theodore Roosevelt's administration and continues even today. Although the Hill-Burton Act required a "reasonable" amount of uncompensated care, it did allow that "non-emergent" care did not qualify under the law's provisions. We also had the creation of Medicare and Medicaid reimbursement in the mid-60s. These legislative actions, combined with the introduction of third-party reimbursement (employer-paid health insurance), inaugurated the modern era of medicine and the diminishing of "comfort care" as a goal of care since virtually every illness was considered curable or such a cure was in sight.

Palliative care is often confused with hospice care. Hospice is for patients with a limited lifespan; it is a service that helps the patient and their loved ones prepare for death. Hospice care is a type of palliative care given to address people's unique needs with terminal illnesses. Unfortunately, palliative care is often considered pain management only to be initiated when other surgical and pharmaceutical methods fail. Palliative care is, in fact, systematic management of the entire range of symptoms that are part of a life-limiting illness when death is not imminent. As Panicola and co-authors point out, "A primary problem is that our health care system pursues two parallel tracks when treating the dying: either an aggressive, curative approach or a comfort care approach."[11] I would add that this parallel approach includes conditions such as heart disease, diabetes, cancer, and COPD that could, with an integrated and coordinated approach, help people live longer and more comfortably. A coordinated approach utilizing palliative care early in the diagnosis would allow for a holistic care plan that addresses the patient's physical, psychological, social, and spiritual needs. It would allow for the discernment process discussed earlier to be fully actualized. As Panicola and co-authors state,

> Palliative care seeks to reclaim the traditional goals of medicine-which, before the advent of modern medical technology, were providing comfort and improving the quality of life-and to integrate these with the more modern goals of curing and prolonging life.[12]

When used correctly, palliative care can work alongside disease management efforts with life-limiting conditions, help manage symptoms, and improve the quality of life when a cure is not currently available and death is not

---

[11] Ibid,180.

[12] Ibid, 181.

looming. We will transform the health care delivery system through an approach that acknowledges and values life's dignity. That is why palliative care is not merely a companion service but is an essential component of health care systems.

Palliative care was first differentiated as a legitimate disciple in England, mainly through Dr. Cicely Saunders' influence. Although Dr. Saunders was primarily concerned with patient needs at the end-of-life, she was instrumental in bringing attention to those patients diagnosed with life-limiting conditions. By the 1970s, palliative care came to be synonymous with the physical, social, psychological, and spiritual support of patients with a life-limiting illness, delivered by a multidisciplinary team. In the U.K. and other European countries, palliative care's specialty or subspecialty was first given official recognition.[13] It was not until 2006, after 14 other countries had done so, that the United States officially recognized palliative care as a subspecialty by the American Board of Medical Specialties.[14]

---

[13] David Clark, "From Margins to Centre: A Review of the History of Palliative Care in Cancer," *The Lancet* 8, no. 5 (May 1, 2007): pp. 430-438, https://doi.org/10.1016/S1470-2045(07)70138-9.

[14] David Clark, "Palliative Medicine as a Specialty," End of Life Studies (University of Glasgow, October 4, 2016), http://endoflifestudies.academicblogs.co.uk/palliative-medicine-as-a-specialty/.

All too often, health care organizations advertise that they have a palliative care service when, in fact, they have only a pain management program in place. The service can be provided in either an inpatient setting or combined with a coordinated outpatient component. There is a certification process an organization can choose to undertake to ensure the program meets the standards for providing the full range of care required for patients with complex medical conditions. The Joint Commission, on its website concerning palliative care services, explains it has a formal certification process that will emphasize to your patients, their families, and your community that your organization has:

- A formally organized inpatient program led by an interdisciplinary team with expertise in palliative care.
- A particular focus on patient and family engagement.
- Processes that support the coordination of care and communication among all care settings and providers.[15]

---

[15] jointcommission.org, https://www.jointcommission.org/accreditation-and-certification/certification/certifications-by-setting/hospital-certifications/palliative-care-certification/

A palliative care service should have a multidisciplinary team that consists of a physician, nurses, including an advanced practice nurse, a social worker, a chaplain, and a pharmacist. Depending on how the program has been organized determines whether all these disciplines are full-time or have designated time as part of their regular schedule. Although this appears to be an expensive program to develop, there are benefits in improved patient outcomes (longer survival rates), patient and family satisfaction, and reduced hospital admissions. Studies indicate cost avoidance (savings) between $3,237 and $4,865 per admission as an incentive to the organization in addition to the other benefits.[16]

I will be discussing the integration of palliative care within what I consider to be a model community hospital in Chapter 9. The critical point I am trying to make in this discussion of palliative care is that it is a prime example of how patients and families can have a voice in choosing how they want to live. It is a service in which a person can make a fully informed decision "to live as well as I can for as long as I can."

---

[16] "The Case for Hospital Palliative Care," *Center to Advance Palliative Care. Center to Advance Palliative Care,* February 25, 2019, https://www.capc.org/toolkits/starting-the-program/designing-an-inpatient-palliative-care-program/.

To complete this section on informed consent, we must also address the end-of-life decision-making process that includes choosing Hospice Care. As I noted earlier, hospice and palliative care are often seen as synonymous terms. I have already noted that palliative care is focused on providing relief from the physical symptoms, spiritual needs, and psychosocial anxiety of life-limiting illness. The goal is to improve the quality of life for both the patient and the family. Palliative care is appropriate at any age and any stage of illness, and it can be provided along with all other medical treatments. The care's beneficial effect is enhancing through earlier engagement with the palliative team and coordination with the patient's primary care team. It does not compete with an existing plan of curative care. Instead, it supports the primary care team's efforts to assist the patient and family in mitigating the patient's suffering.

As I indicated, palliative and hospice care are often used as interchangeable terms because both provide what is termed "comfort care." The objective of both is to reduce worry and offer complex symptom relief related to a serious illness—both palliative and hospice care address physical and psychosocial relief for patients. Palliative care is for those seeking curative treatment simultaneously. Hospice care is for those with a prognosis of six months or less who do not seek curative treatment or are no longer responding to the procedures or medications. It can be initiated when two physicians certify that the patient has fewer than six months to live if the illness follows its predictable course. It is comfort care without curative intent. The patient is no longer responding to restorative treatment or has elected not to continue nonbeneficial treatments. Unlike palliative care, which is often reimbursed on a fee-for-service basis like other health care services, hospice services are covered by Medicare, Medicaid, and most private insurance. It is most often a service that is delivered in a home setting or a nursing home. The service duration can be months, weeks, or just a few days (most commonly occurring in a hospital). Hospice emphasizes care rather than cure. The goal is to provide comfort during the final months and days of life.

Fortunately, the average length of time in hospice has gradually increased to a 2019 average of over 71 days. In addition, 98% of the care is provided outside a hospital setting. Hospice length of stay in hospitals is less than one week and is often merely an administrative disposition when all treatment options have been exhausted. That means the patient and family have often been put into a stressful situation in which the discernment process discussed earlier is not possible. Decisions are made primarily out of emotion and often result in ethics consultations to address the provider and patient/family conflict. Often advance care planning has not taken place. There has been no consultation with the palliative care team in the disease process. All too often, nonbeneficial (expensive) procedures are tried as a defensive measure to avoid claims that "everything" was not attempted to save the patient. My experience in these situations is that they are the most frequent initiators of a clinical ethics consultation and can set the stage for unnecessary conflict between the patient/family and providers.

In their report entitled *Dying in America: Improving Quality and Honoring Individual Preferences Near the End of Life*, the *Institute of Medicine of the National Academies* points out that people nearing the end of life frequently experience multiple transitions between health care settings.[17] This frequent relocation would include high rates of apparently preventable hospitalizations. Recurrent relocation introduces confusion with the delivery of care since unaffiliated organizations often provide care. This fragmentation creates burdens for patients and families. Families have often been put into the caregivers' position— something for which they may have little to no training. By introducing palliative care early in the disease process, data indicates "a higher quality of life, including better understanding and communication, access to home care, emo-

---

[17] Committee on Approaching Death: Addressing Key End of Life Issues, "The Delivery of Person-Centered, Family-Oriented End-of-Life Care." *Dying in America: Improving Quality and Honoring Individual Preferences Near the End of Life*, (U.S. National Library of Medicine, March 19, 2015), https://www.ncbi.nlm.nih.gov/books/NBK285676/.

tional and spiritual support, well-being and dignity, care at the time of death, and lighter symptom burden."[18]

While the evidence is not definitive, there is a sense that palliative care and hospice patients may live longer than similarly ill patients who do not receive such care. Although the practice of routinely asking for a palliative consult for patients with a life-limiting illness is not yet universal, the training of physicians, along with the positive results of early referral, is encouraging. I will discuss in Chapter 9 how one program went from pain management for patients near the end–of-life to a fully integrated element of the inpatient care protocols in a matter of a few months.

Summary

Previous chapters discussed freedom and virtuous living. Both of these concepts are components of the discussion concerning informed consent. This chapter focuses on informed consent's central importance, allowing one to make reasoned decisions for those with a life-limiting illness. Note, I did not say end-of-life, although that is undoubtedly a factor to be addressed. Informed consent is directed at allowing the individual to flourish within the opportunities available to them. The conversation also in-

---

[18] Ibid.

vestigated the roles of family and friends in supporting and enhancing the community of love in which each of us lives.

The chapter has also addressed the desirability of having a medical home and advanced care plan created in cooperation with a person trained to help people express their wishes. It has also discussed palliative care's appropriateness as part of the care plan for those diagnosed with a life-limiting illness.

Suggested Reading

https://respectingchoices.org/ is the website that gives an overview of advance care planning's approach that has been successfully introduced throughout the United States and several other countries. The program originated in La Crosse, Wisconsin, under Bud Hammes' leadership.

Health Care Ethics: A Catholic Theological Analysis, authored by Benedict Ashley, O.P., Jean deBlois, C.S.J., and Kevin O'Rourke, O.P. These three were instrumental in establishing the Health Care Ministry program at the Aquinas Institute of Theology in St. Louis, Missouri.

An Introduction to Health Care Ethics, Theological Foundations, Contemporary Issues, and Controversial Cases, by Michael Panicola, David Belde, John Paul Slosar, and Mark Repenshek, a valuable introduction to health care ethics. The book provides foundational theology and philosophy for health care ethics.

Palliative Care and Catholic Health Care: Two Millennia of Caring for the Whole Person, edited by Peter J. Cataldo and Dan O'Brien, is a comprehensive overview of the compatibility of palliative care with the vision of human dignity. It is a resource on palliative care, including care at the end of life, for bioethicists, theologians, and palliative care specialists; other health care professionals, can also benefit from its contents. Health care sponsors, administrators and executives, clergy, students, and patients receiving palliative care and their families will also find this book a clarifying and reassuring resource.

https//: www.capc.org is the website address for the Center to Advance Palliative Care. The site provides the information necessary to help healthcare providers establish "best practices" palliative care programs.

Chapter Eight

Faith-Based Health Care

Our LORD Jesus Christ,
Suffering in the multitude
Of sick and infirm of every kind,
seeks relief at your hands.
(Bishop Claude Dubuis, 1866)

The emphasis so far has been on living a virtuous life from an individual and, to some extent, a community perspective. From this point on, the focus will be on how, in particular, faith-based Catholic health care organizations can not only participate but also be the catalyst that enables those within the community served to flourish. Faith-based health care services are not the exclusive domain of Catholic organizations but represent the most extensive health-care delivery system. I have personally worked with Baptist, Lutheran, Presbyterian, Episcopal, Seventh Day Adventist, Methodist, Jewish, and Mormon health care organizations during my career. I include this chapter because it is critical to understand the history behind faith-based organizations' efforts to help communities flourish.

What makes Catholic health care organizations unique is their numbers and the fidelity each must maintain to Church teaching and authority to retain their identity as Catholic organizations. The Catholic Health Association reports that as of 2020, there are 668 hospitals and 1,666 long-term care and other health facilities members in all 50 states. The Catholic health ministry is the largest group of nonprofit health care providers in the United States. It is estimated that one in six patients in the U.S. is cared for in a Catholic hospital. These numbers account for only a portion of Catholic health care worldwide, including over 5,500 hospitals; 65% are in developing countries.[1]

Although Catholic health care organizations are divided into many large systems, they are united in their adherence to the Catholic Church's teaching. This faithfulness to the Church's teaching is outlined in a document entitled *Ethical and Religious Directives for Catholic Health Care Services* (ERDs), now in its sixth edition. The document states:

The purpose of these Ethical and Religious Directives then is twofold: first, to reaffirm the ethical standards of behavior in health care that flow from the Church's teaching about the dignity of the human person; sec-

---

[1] "Catholic Health Care in America," *Facts - Statistics* (Catholic Health Association, January 2020), https://chausa.org/about/about/facts-statistics.

ond, to provide authoritative guidance on certain moral issues that face Catholic health care today.[2]

The ERDs, as they are commonly referred to, are used to express the Church's moral teaching. They serve to guide leaders, providers of care at all levels, and patients/families within Catholic health care organizations. The Table of Contents for the document outlines the comprehensive nature of the Bishops' direction in consultation with theologians, ethicists, and providers. The document deals with social responsibility, an obligation to provide spiritual care, instruction on demonstrating mutual respect, trust, honesty, and appropriate confidentiality in the provider-patient relationship. The document is probably best known and most controversial for its straight-forward commitment to life from its natural beginning to a natural end. The text concludes with guidance on serving the common good, specifically in collaboration with various non-Catholic partners. The document clarifies that such collaboration cannot be condoned if the partner is an organization that does not conform to the Church's moral teaching. The ERDs then provide us with a clear view of how the institu-

---

[2] *Ethical and Religious Directives for Catholic Health Care Services* (Washington, D.C., DC: United States Conference of Catholic Bishops, 2018), 1-2.

tional Church hierarchy sees Catholic health care as not merely a subsidiary but a partner in the ministry.

Providing care, including formal health care services, is not a 20th-century invention of the Church. As part of the ministry of Jesus Christ, healing has always been central to the expression of God's mercy and love for creation. Jesus instructed his followers to heal the sick (Lk 9:1-2; Mk 16:15-18; Mt 10:8). The early Christians were noted for tending the sick and infirm. The Christian emphasis on practical charity gave rise to systematic nursing and hospitals' development. In the early Church, a minority religion, we had the development of processes to assist those in need. Acts 6:1-6 describes how the new ministry of service for the community was differentiated from the preaching by the institution of the office of *Diakonos*, a Greek word meaning servant. The persons chosen were to perform acts of service for the community. It must be noted that the issue that precipitated the establishment of the diaconate was a question of just distribution among the various groups of widows (Hellenists and Hebrews). In time, we see ways to assist the poor, deal with abandoned children, and even develop nascent hospitals.

The healing stories given in the Gospels have served as the impetus for the development of health care services among all Christian denominations. Catholic health care also sees the parable of the Good Samaritan as foundational. Dan O'Brien notes the parable is in answer to the question *And who is my neighbor* (Lk 10:29). O'Brien points out that scholars spend much energy trying to understand the motivation for each of the characters' actions. He argues that the story is one in which Jesus teaches his listeners to have compassion for our perceived enemies.[3] The story has been seen as an allegorical interpretation in which the Samaritan represents Jesus, who shows compassion for all.

Fr. Gerald Arbuckle writes that in the opinion of St. John Paul II, "The parable that best articulated the heart of the health care mission and ministry of Jesus Christ was that of the Good Samaritan."[4] He further notes that in the encyclical *Deus Caritas Est,* Pope Benedict XVI points four times to the significance of the Good Samaritan parable as the model for holistic care."[5] Arbuckle identifies the story as containing several forms of violence, including verbal, physical, social, ritual, racial, and occupational. His interpretation of the parable emphasizes how one can respond

---

[3] Dan O'Brien, "Palliative Care and the Catholic Healing Ministry: Biblical and Historical Roots," in *Palliative Care and Catholic Health Care: Two Millennia of Caring for the Whole Person,* ed. Peter J. Cataldo and Dan O'Brien (Cham, Switzerland: Springer, 2019), pp. 9-24.

[4] Gerald Arbuckle, "Retelling the Good Samaritan'" (*Catholic Health Association,* 2007), https://www.chausa.org/publications/health-progress/article/july-august-2007/retelling-the-good-samaritan

[5] Ibid.

to violence with compassion and justice. He connects the Samaritan actions with values and actions fundamental to Catholic health, such as seeing the dignity in each person, a preference for those who are powerless, and proper use of those resources available in service to your neighbor. He also accentuates how the Samaritan's action helped bring the victim back into his community. All of these (and several others) are essential characteristics for those organizations that wish to identify as Catholic. A thorough review of what a Catholic identity means will follow in this chapter.

Before leaving this section, I wish to discuss the Good Samaritan parable (Lk 10:25-37) as a foundational story for Catholic health care. I want to show how I used this story as an example for new associates at CHRISTUS St. Michael Health System. During orientation, we devoted several hours looking at the question, "What makes us Catholic?" This interpretation was an essential concern in that less than 3% of the new associates identified as being of the Catholic faith. However, virtually all the associates would self-identify as either Christian and belonging to a particular denomination.

With all due respect to Dan O'Brien's comment on the inordinate energy devoted to analyzing the characters' motivation, I found it useful to compare each of the characters to parallel situations we see in the workplace—specifically the health care ministry. I characterized the lawyer as the person in the workgroup who likes to play "gotcha" by asking a seemingly innocent question with the hope of trapping someone into making a statement that could be portrayed maliciously or provocatively. The Priest and the Levite could, with justification, show that their other responsibilities precluded them from approaching the victim. The victim is irresponsible in his action of journeying alone on what was known to be a dangerous road. The robbers can be seen as disadvantaged people and only taking what was due them. The point being made was that taking positions that avoided responsibility for living the organization's values and mission is often available in the workplace. That is, we can justify our actions in light of our desires and perceived needs.

I would then contrast the story's characters with the Samaritan and the innkeeper. The Samaritan lived under the same ritual purity rules as the Priest and Levite; he had no obligation to serve the unknown victim (he was stripped and thus unidentifiable), who could have been an enemy. The innkeeper (recognize that innkeepers were often seen as unfair) was entrusted to provide proper care for the victim. There was enough trust that the Samaritan was willing to pay any additional amount beyond his initial deposit to assure the victim received what he needed. I then asked, "Who are we in the parable?" Invariably, the new Associates would make us the heroes of the story—the Samaritan. My response was, "No, we are the innkeeper." We are the ones seen as being only in it for the money, uncaring, large, impenetrable bureaucracies whose concern was reputation and market share.

In my telling of the story (with apologies to real scholars), the central point was the Sisters founded the ministry on a platform of care, compassion, dignity, and love for one's neighbor. The question is answered in Luke's parable with the reply to Jesus' question: *Which of these three, do you think, proved to be a neighbor to the man who fell among the robbers? He said, "The one who showed him mercy." And Jesus said to him, "You go, and do likewise* (Lk 10:36-37). We then must ask, "Are we the ones who show mercy?"

During the Middle Ages, monasteries and convents were the key medical centers of Europe, and the Church developed an early version of a welfare state. It was in these locations that key medical findings were achieved because they were focused on education. Catholic institutions of higher learning (Cathedral schools) advanced into a network of medieval universities. Catholic scientists (many of them clergymen) made many important discoveries that aided modern science and medical development. For instance, Gregor Mendel, an Augustinian priest, initially developed theories on genetics. Ironically, many of the advancements in medicine were derived from Islamic physicians. Europeans then appropriated these practices as "takeaways" from the period of the Crusades.

The hospital concept was emerging in parts of the Roman Empire in the 4th century. These were specialized facilities where people could be treated by individuals trained in the healing arts. The original hospitals began in the early Christian communities to provide lodging and care for the poor and travelers. In the Christian areas, hospitals were typically run by monasteries and gradually became more extensive and more complex over the Middle Ages. With the advancement in medical knowledge (influenced by Islamic medical practices), the Latin and Byzantine world began to see illness as physical problems that could be successfully treated instead of seeing sin as the cause of disease.

Before the Reformation Period (16th-17th centuries), it was religious orders of men that were most actively engaged in providing hospitals. Up to that point, most religious women lived in cloistered communities. This way of living changed again in the 18th and 19th centuries as more and more religious communities of women were founded, with many having a "charism" (a gift that flows from God's love to humanity) for caring for the sick. Caring for the sick once again became a common vocation among women in religious communities. When these religious groups came to the United States, hospitals were among the institutions that they founded.

The specific task of many of these groups of women was to care for the sick poor. Education and health care became the hallmarks of these congregations. Often, the hospitals founded by these religious communities served dual purposes. They served where there was discrimination against Catholic immigrants. Just as crucial in terms of the mission was that Catholic hospitals were open to all. They provided for both the medical and the spiritual needs of their patients. They were inclusive (before the term was fashionable) by allowing Protestant clergy to visit patients even though Catholic clergy were often not welcome in many public or private hospitals.

This practice of care for the poor is still seen as a priority in Catholic health care. It is expressed in the mission statements and the lists of core values that are now part of Catholic health care. There is an expression of preference for the poor in delivering accessible health care services in these mission statements. For Catholic health care, access to care is an issue of distributive justice, especially resource allocation to serve vulnerable populations. Catholic health care emphasizes human dignity, care for the poor, the sacredness of life, service, integrity, justice, and compassion. The various Catholic health care systems' mission and vision statements nearly always convey that the system's work participates in Christ's healing ministry.

The story of the Catholic Sisters from the various religious communities is often quite similar. I will use the founding of the American ministry of the Sisters of Charity of the Incarnate Word as an example. In full disclosure, my experience as a Mission Leader in Catholic health care was within an organization initially sponsored by the Sisters of Charity of the Incarnate Word, Houston Congregation. Their account represents many other religious congregations' courage in leaving their homes (most often in Europe) to come to America to serve God. The Sisters' story is well-documented in CHRISTUS St. Michael Health Systems Anniversary celebration book, *100 Years of Healing*.[6]

The story of the founding of the Sisters of Charity of the Incarnate Word represents how religious women and men endured significant difficulties in their effort to serve the LORD in a health ministry. The story begins with Bishop Dubuis, the second Bishop of Galveston, which included all of Texas, who had arrived in the United States as a French missionary in 1844. He was appointed Bishop of Texas in 1862. Texas was a vast area for one person to serve. Moreover, Texas had many poor people as a result of the aftermath of the Civil War. It had experienced overwhelming outbreaks of cholera and yellow fever.

In 1866, Dubuis appealed to his friend Mother Angelique, Superior of the Order of the Incarnate Word and

---

[6] *100 Years of Healing* is a commemorative book created by the communications department of CHRISTUS St. Michael health System. It tells the Sisters of Incarnate Word founding story and how they established a ministry in Texarkana. An electronic copy can be accessed at http://christusstmichael.org/100years, 9.

Blessed Sacrament in Lyons, France. The Order had been founded in the early part of the 17th century by Jeanne Chezard de Matel. Texas was not unknown to the Sisters since, at the request of the first Bishop of Galveston, John Mary Odin, C.M., the Order's members had been sent to Brownsville. Sisters from this Order subsequently established educational institutions in several other Texas communities as early as 1853. Bishop Dubuis again turned to the Sisters seeking assistance, saying in his letter to them, "Our LORD Jesus Christ, suffering in the persons of a multitude of the sick and infirm of every kind, seeks relief at your hands."[7]

Mother Angelique could not fulfill his request since the community was cloistered and was committed to the ministry of education for youth. Bishop Dubuis then requested the admission of three young women from Lyon, who had volunteered. They were received into the community to accept formation and the rule of the Order. It was understood from the beginning that a new Congregation was being formed. A Congregation was different from the cloistered Order of the Incarnate Word and Blessed Sacrament. It was intentionally established to be dedicated to active service work for the Church in health care.

These three young women accepted the call to begin a new ministry in Texas. On September 23, 1866, the three

---

[7] Ibid.

received the habit (the distinctive garb that acted as an outward sign of consecration to God) of the new Congregation. Their names were Sister Mary Blandine Mathelin, Sister Mary Joseph Roussin, and Sister Mary Ange Escude. Two days later, they left on a treacherous sea voyage to Texas in which they had to endure high seas and a hurricane. By April of 1867, they opened St. Mary's Infirmary in Galveston. It was the first Catholic hospital in Texas. Unfortunately, in that same year, within a few months of the hospital's opening, a yellow fever epidemic struck Galveston. The outbreak was devastating for the population and resulted in Sister Mary Blandine's death. Sister Mary Ange, who had recovered from the illness, had to return to France. Fortunately, other women joined the congregation, and the Sisters' ministry expanded throughout Texas and adjoining states. A second Congregation was founded in 1869 in San Antonio as a sister house of the Sisters of Charity of the Incarnate Word, Galveston, Texas. Both Congregations created successful health care ministries as well as expanded their charism to include education. The Galveston Congregation later moved to Houston to ultimately establish a presence in what is today named CHRISTUS St. Michael Health System.

St. Michael Hospital was not the first such facility in Texarkana. In the early part of the 20th century, the 4 States area (Texas, Arkansas, Louisiana, and Oklahoma) had limited availability of care for the poor. At that time, a local

Irish-Catholic named Michael Meagher, a civil engineer, and community leader died. He left an estate of $75,000 for the express intent to "erect a charity hospital for the treatment of all poor and indigent persons in need of medical attention" (excerpted from Mr. Meagher's will).[8]

The will explicitly directed the trustees to the estate to find a suitable lot in or near the City of Texarkana to build a charity hospital. The book, *100 Years of Healing*, created by CHRISTUS St. Michael Health System, provides information taken from "Serving from Gladness," the history of the Congregation written by Sr. Mary Loyola Hegarty, CCVI, which relates:

> In 1915, Mother Teresea O'Gara, CCVI, and the Council of the Congregation of the Sisters of Charity of the Incarnate Word (Houston Congregation) accepted an offer from the Board of Trustees of the estate of Michael Meagher to lease and operate a hospital for indigent sick in Texarkana, Arkansas, a proposal that had been offered by the Board the previous year.[9]

The original location was a renovated former hospital. It was to be operated by the Sisters under a 25-year lease arrangement. During the time of renovation, Sr. Sacred

---

[8] Ibid, 11.

[9] Ibid, 10.

Heart Travers and Sr. Mary Clare McDonnell lived in the home of P. J. Ahern, the person who had negotiated the lease arrangement on behalf of the Trustees. At the time, prejudice against Catholics was not unusual, and thus, the fact that the Aherns allowed the sisters to live in their home was a remarkable act of courage.

The hospital's first patient's story is legendary and re-markably consistent with the mission that the Sisters ac-cepted. The story is told that Phillip Brooks, a transient with neither money nor a job, was the first patient. He was found dying in the hospital's boiler room on the very day it was to open.[10] Mr. Brooks was the model of the typical pa-tient the hospital was designed to serve. To this day, the hospital is seen within the community as the "safety net" for underserved and vulnerable people. While I became the Vice President of Mission Integration for CHRISTUS St. Michael Health System in 2011, it was not my first hospital experience.

In the early 1980's, the then St. Michael Hospital, which was part of the Sisters of Charity of the Incarnate Word, Houston Congregation's hospital system, hired the compa-ny I worked for to manage what we then called an "alcohol-ism treatment unit" (CAREunit). St. Michael's became one of the locations with which I became quite familiar, as the

---

[10] Ibid, 13.

hospital administrator was a member of the Congregation with a well-deserved formidable reputation.

Sr. Carmelita Brett had been assigned to lead St. Michael at a time in its history when there was some question about the ability to continue the ministry in Texarkana. Dr. Tom Alston, a medical staff leader, reminisced that the hospital was in severe financial distress throughout the 1960s because of its free care to the poor. This practice was commonplace before Medicare and Medicaid programs were fully operational (both were enacted into law in the mid-1960s). Dr. Alston characterized Sr. Carmelita as one who had a "commanding force about her."[11] Dr. Alston, as well as many others, credited her with turning things around for the hospital. She was able to accomplish the revitalization of the ministry by instituting sound business practices. Sister Carmelita restructured the governing board as a public body to attract key people and organizations within Texarkana to see the hospital as a community asset rather than simply being owned by the Sisters. She also embarked on recruiting new physicians, particularly in specialty areas that were not well represented. Her stewardship strategy allowed the hospital to remain viable and prepared for developing a modern campus that enabled the organization to become a leader in Texarkana and gain national prominence.

---

[11] Ibid, 45.

At the same time that I had the privilege of working with Sr. Carmelita, I was also fortunate enough to also work with other religious congregations of women. These leaders belonged to congregations like Daughters of Charity, Sisters of Mercy, and Sisters of Charity of Leavenworth. These women were not only leaders in their industry but would have been successful in running giant corporations. One thing Sr. Carmelita emphasized to me was loyalty. That is, Sister committed to working with our company to assure the success of the program; she, in turn, made it clear that she wanted a commitment from me that the company I represented would be faithful to St. Michael's mission. Sr. Carmelita's relationship with everyone, including the senior management of the company I worked for, was respected because it was built on a foundation of honesty, integrity, and justice. Sr. Carmelita was the last member of her Congregation to be the Chief Executive Officer of St. Michael Hospital. She established a foundation on which subsequent leaders could build. While she was the last religious Sister who was CEO, St. Michael continued to have Sisters from the Houston Congregation and Benedictine nuns who served in the hospital as Chaplains. Even today, as many health care ministries no longer have active Sisters, CHRISTUS St. Michael continues to have sisters from the Houston congregation and a member of the Society of the Sacred Heart.

I related in the opening of this book how I came to be appointed as the Vice President of Mission Integration. I was to succeed Sr. Damian Murphy, an important figure in St. Michael's history. Sr. Damian had held several positions over the years as she was trained as a Registered Nurse, administrator, chaplain, and ethicist. From 1985 until her retirement in 2010, she was Director of Pastoral Care and, ultimately, Vice President of Mission Integration. This leadership is a role that is found almost exclusively in Catholic health care. It is a function that began developing in the late 1970s as the number of nuns in health care began to diminish. Up to that time, the definition of a Catholic hospital was "ones that had nuns." Like many Catholic hospitals at one time or another, St. Michael had Sisters playing leading clinical and administrative roles in every department. Being filled by a Sister, the mission integration function became the organization's visible identification as Catholic. Their responsibilities revolved around managing pastoral care and dealing with questions involving clinical and organizational ethics. They were the "moral compass" of the organization.

To illustrate what I mean, I would like to relate two events that happened to me during the hiring process. First, I was asked to participate in a telephone interview with the administrative team before an in-person interview. This interview process taking place before the video conference was such a common practice. The meeting lasted for approximately 1 hour, after which I spoke with Chris Karam, the CEO. My initial question was that I had heard the people report, "Sr. Damian said," several times. I was surprised she had asked me no questions. Chris paused and then said, "Sr. Damian has been gone for six months." My reply was, "Sr. Damian is still in that room." The point is that the administrative team had been reliant upon the sisters such as Sr. Damian to be their "Catholic identity." I was now the first "layperson" to serve in the role of mission leader in an organization that was still dependent on Sr. Damian's guidance.

The second event occurred when I attended mass at the Catholic Church in which Sr. Damian had been a member. After the service, the Pastor introduced me as the person taking Sr. Damian's place. There was an audible gasp. Nancy Keenan, the Chief Nursing Executive at CHRISTUS St. Michael, and I talked about that event later as an example of how much Sr. Damian had meant to the community. Fortunately, the foundation that Sr. Damian had set was more deeply embedded than the administrative team recognized. Sr. Damian, Sr. Carmelita, and all the other Sisters who had served the ministry over the years had planted the seeds within the Texarkana community that were now bearing the fruit.

St. Michael became part of the aptly named CHRISTUS Health System by combining the health care ministries of the two Sisters of Charity of the Incarnate Word congregations in 1999. A third sponsoring congregation, the Sisters of the Holy Family of Nazareth, joined in 2016. When I joined CHRISTUS St. Michael in 2011, the corporate entity operated in three locations to provide organizational support. The Houston location was primarily administrative functions, and the San Antonio location was information technology. Dallas was where executive leadership was officed. Eventually, the advantages of having a centralized corporate headquarters were recognized. Thus, in 2015, the corporate headquarters were established in the Irving, Texas suburb of Dallas.

As noted above, CHRISTUS Health is sponsored by the Sisters of Charity of the Incarnate Word in Houston and San Antonio and The Sisters of the Holy Family of Nazareth. These organizations are entities formally sanctioned by church authority carried out publicly under its auspices. These religious congregations are organized as a health care ministry to guarantee CHRISTUS Health's continuation as Catholic. The Sisters from the congregations retain seats on the organization's governing body and retain certain reserved rights, such as approving the system's CEO. The purpose of this type of governing structure was to assure that the ministries established by these religious congregations would be able to continue to exist in the new world of complex business arrangements and substantial capital requirements. The Sisters had prepared the way for the ministry's continuation, much as Jesus had prepared his disciples to continue. Although many Catholic health care organizations no longer have nuns in executive positions, they continue to have the legacy and spiritual influence that these religious congregations provided and continue contributing to the ministries they founded.

Catholic identity is a term that many throughout Catholic health care would have difficulty defining. It was easy to say you were Catholic if your CEO was a nun or religious Brother/Priest, and others of your Congregation were serving critical functions in the organization. I remember one of my Aquinas classmates' responses to the question, "How do you know your hospital is Catholic?" This person was not Catholic and worked in a non-Catholic hospital recently acquired by a Catholic entity. He answered, "Because we have nuns." That was an unusual response since his location had no nun in any positions and never had a nun working in the facility. His identification as Catholic was not dependent on how the organization conducted business but because it had representatives of a religious congregation. Another example of the ubiquitous nature of that definition of being Catholic can also be heard when people say, "This place (usually a hospital) is sure different without the nuns." In other words, there is the perception, real or imagined, that the Sisters were less interested in prudent business practices and more in providing free care. As I noted earlier, my experience with religious Sisters in administrative positions is that they were thoroughly familiar with operational effectiveness and the need for both stewardship and charity (love). The issue was how do we, as the new leaders in Catholic health care, retain the ability to serve as a ministry without the visible presence of those who had been the icons of Catholic health care?

Another component of the transition from leadership principally coming from within the religious Congregation was the relationship with the bishops. To be considered Catholic means the organization must be in communion with the Church and its leadership. In this case, the Bishop of the diocese in which the facility is located is the leader to whom the local health system leader responds. Still, most large Catholic health care organizations have locations in multiple dioceses. Thus, there is no one central authority. Second, the bishop and the religious often had mutual respect relationships because both parties have demonstrated a commitment to a life serving God through the Church and the willing sacrifices each makes in pursuit of their vocations.

Moreover, both parties knew the rules and intentions of the Church. An implicit level of trust existed, even in times of disagreement. That same level of trust did not always exist with lay leadership, some of whom were not Catholic. Therefore, this new type of leadership task was to establish the bishop's trust level and continue the Sister's legacy of prudent business practices, which included charity in a demonstrated manner.

Maintaining a Catholic identity brings me back to the story I told at the beginning of this book about a meeting that Sr. Jean Connell, CCVI, Latin for *Congregatio Caritatis Verbi Incarnati,* Fr. Lawrence Chellaian, Director of Spiritual Care, Chris Karam, CEO, and I had with Bishop Taylor in 2012. At that time, the Bishop was engaged in a difference of opinion with a Catholic health system in the process of selling one of its hospitals in Arkansas to a for-profit entity. One of the local hospital board members who resigned over the issue is quoted in the October 12, 2012, edition of the *St. Louis Post-Dispatch* as saying, "A lot of things changed when the sisters stopped running the system and turned it over to the lay leaders. The new approach is the Almighty Dollar." Bishop Taylor, in the same article, is quoted as calling the action "a decision to sell …. an abandonment of the ministry." Ultimately, the Bishop and the health system in question were able to resolve the issue by selling the property to another Catholic health care organization operating within Arkansas. The controversy was occurring at the time of our meeting with the Bishop.

As I noted earlier, the Bishop was very cordial, although he did ask one surprising question: "Did we travel to Little Rock by air?" Chris Karam, who is known for his wit and quick thinking, answered, "No, but we did come in one Accord." That was true. We had traveled from Texarkana in a 2005 Honda Accord Hybrid, which had been donated to the hospital and at that time had nearly 180,000 miles on the odometer. Bishop Taylor did not respond to Chris's amusing response, signaling that this would be a serious meeting. As I indicated earlier, Bishop Taylor's question concerning what makes us Catholic penetrated us to our core, both individually and as an organization. It was clear that we had seen our good works and acting as a self-defined, safety-net hospital as evidence that we were a Catholic, faith-based organization. Now it was incumbent upon us to discern who we were as an entity that we called Catholic. This meeting initiated a discernment process spoken of in Chapter 7 that included the virtue of prudence and the involvement of a spiritual component, including introspection. It contemplates organizational thoughts, desires, and conduct combined with reason, allowing informed decisions resulting in personal and corporate flourishing. The discernment process included engaging and actively listening to health care providers and the community to be served. We believed such engagement was necessary to have an integrated and health-focused system with a clear Catholic identity.

Adding to the urgency, we now felt a need to differentiate our health system from a secular health care provider due to an investigation completed by Sandra Hapenney concerning adherence to Church teaching by Catholic hospitals regarding elective sterilization. Hapenney is a resident scholar at Baylor University's Institute for Studies of

Religion.[12] Hapenney, using 2008 publicly available health data, had studied hospitals throughout Texas and discovered that a significant number of Catholic hospitals in Texas allowed tubal ligation. This finding was taken very seriously by Bishop Alvaro Corrada of the Diocese of Tyler. He addressed the issue at two offending hospitals within his jurisdiction by banning all such procedures. Tyler is the diocese in which CHRISTUS St. Michael is located and was thus subject to this strict interpretation of the Ethical and Religious Directives.

The point in discussing the requirements placed upon Catholic hospitals in the Diocese of Tyler is not to debate the Church's teaching. In the recommended readings, I will offer viewpoints from both sides of the issue. The ERDs have language that addresses sterilization,

> Direct sterilization of either men or women, whether permanent or temporary, is not permitted in a Catholic health care institution. Procedures that induce sterility are permitted when their direct effect in the cure or alleviation of a present and serious pathology and a sim-

---

[12] "Half of US Catholic Hospitals Do Sterilizations, Report Suggests: News Headlines," (*Catholic World News*, February 12, 2012), https://www.catholicculture.org/news/headlines/index.cfm?storyid=13400.

pler treatment is not available (ERD, Part 5, Directive 53).[13]

We were aware that any effort we undertook to demonstrate our Catholic identity must consider Bishop Corrada and his successor, Bishop Joseph Strickland's, position on many issues. They were interested in not just sterilization but all our clinical and business practices.

We were fortunate that identifying CHRISTUS Health as a Catholic organization was of utmost concern to CHRISTUS Health leadership's upper levels. Ernie Sadau, CEO, Gerry Heeley, Executive Vice President of Mission Integration, and the sponsoring congregations of the Sisters of Charity of the Incarnate Word and The Sisters of the Holy Family of Nazareth were all resolved to assure the legacy of the Sisters would be continued. Gerry Heeley had been actively interviewing organizations that might be able to provide the CHRISTUS ministries with an objective analysis of the strengths and opportunities for improvement that each ministry had regarding their fidelity to CHRISTUS Health's mission of "extending the healing ministry of Jesus Christ."

The evaluation tool chosen was the Catholic Identity Matrix (CIM) that was the product of a collaboration between Ascension Health and the University of St. Thomas,

---

[13] *Ethical and Religious Directives*, 24.

Opus College of Business (formerly known as the SAIP Institute). The CIM was developed in response to Ascension Health's (the largest Catholic health care organization) desire to have a method of assessing the ministry's faithfulness to its mission. It was first used in 2006 within Ascension and has since expanded to serve many Catholic health systems nationally and internationally. The CIM facilitates an assessment of Catholic health care organizations in light of six principles: solidarity with the poor, holistic care, respect for human life and dignity, participatory community of work and mutual respect, common good/stewardship, and acting in communion with the Church. It uses a model similar to the Malcolm Baldridge award using self-assessment to help organizations assess whether an organization uses an effective and efficient approach for running the organization, consistent with its stated purpose.

With its self-assessment approach, the CIM was an ideal fit for CHRISTUS St. Michael. We had already applied to and gained the American Nurses Credentialing Center's (ANCC) Magnet Recognition Program®. Besides, we had involvement with our successful application and recognition with the Quality Texas Award. The Quality Texas Foundation promotes the use of the Baldrige Criteria for Performance Excellence and other methods that drive efficiency and effectiveness. CHRISTUS St. Michael volunteered to be the first ministry in the system to undertake the self-assessment based upon the experience in successfully undertaking quality initiatives similar to the CIM. The organization then began a process that lasted approximately 8-months to prepare for the interview process carried out by the CIM facilitators.

CHRISTUS St. Michael's leadership took advantage of the opportunity to be the first applicant for the CIM in the system for several reasons. First, based on Bishops Corrada and Taylor's feedback, we were confident in our ability to serve as a Church ministry. Although it may have appeared that both had been critical of our ministry, both appreciated and respected the willingness we had to speak candidly and directly to the issue of Catholic identity. We maintained that good working relationship with Bishop Joseph Strickland, who succeeded Bishop Corrada after the latter's assignment to a diocese in Puerto Rico. Bishop Strickland was from the Diocese of Tyler and had been our primary contact with the diocesan office.

The second reason for our confidence was the response we had received from surveys of the local community and our associates; we were seen as an excellent place to work and the preferred health care provider. We had been named the Best Place to Work in Texarkana and the State of Texas numerous times. In fact, in 2010, CHRISTUS St. Michael was named Best Place to Work in Health Care by *Modern Healthcare* magazine. We were recognized for the Quality Texas Foundation and named a 100 Top Hospital by IBM Watson Health™ two times (see Appendix A). The point is, we believed we were prepared for an extensive review based on the body of work that had been accumulated over 20 years.

The third reason we chose to volunteer for the process was a sincere desire on the part of the leadership team to undertake an accounting of how we were committed to our founders' legacy and faithful to the mission "to extend the healing ministry of Jesus Christ." Chris Karam was primarily motivated since, for the first time since he had been named President and CEO in 2003, he did not have a member of the founding Congregation in a senior leadership position. Chris had great respect for nuns and priests. He had also been associated with the Sisters of Charity of the Incarnate Word in various healthcare system positions before becoming CEO. Chris was extremely conscious of the heritage we had been gifted and dedicated to building on that foundation. His desire was not merely being a 100 Top Hospital; he wanted to be a mission-driven hospital and thereby show that one could be a ministry that acted out of prudence, compassion, charity, and stewardship.

A final reason was that being the first within the system to take on the process meant there were no preexisting expectations. We believed we would have more latitude to pursue our primary goals to assess how we stood in relationship with fidelity to the mission and identify areas we could improve.

Two difficult tasks had to be completed before having
the CIM facilitators visit. First, we had to organize the
enormous volume of data and policies accumulated in operating a health care organization in a highly regulated industry. Fortunately, we had the work completed in the
Magnet designation and the Quality Texas Foundation application process. Nancy Keenan, Chief Nursing Officer,
and Sue Johnson, Director of Advocacy and Community
Planning, were invaluable in assuring that all the information needed was made available. The second formidable
task was selecting team members to serve on the Catholic
health care workgroup's various principles. Each workgroup consisted of six to eight members capable of evaluating how successfully these principles are embedded in the
operating policies and processes. It was difficult to pare
down the list of potential candidates due to the workforce's
many remarkable candidates. Of course, that was a good
problem to have.

As I noted earlier, the organization entered into the
process with the confidence we were doing "many good
things already." Our purpose was to identify what the CIM
folks called "Opportunities for Improvement." The evaluation process's result was that the CIM team reported that
our ministry had scored higher than any previously surveyed organization. Moreover, there was a high degree of
consistency within each of the principles. That is, we scored
well within each principle. That feedback was gratifying,

demonstrating that the organization was serious about serving as a Church ministry. The process also illuminated two critical areas in which improvement was both necessary and possible. The first had to do with our process of documenting what we did. The survey showed that we engaged in many activities consistent with our mission, but we did them without documenting the action. We were too dependent on single or small groups of Associates to sustain a particular process. To put it in terms of living virtuously, we were not taking good situational habits exhibited by a select group and expanding them to what we internally called "hardwired" policy applicable to the entire ministry.

The second issue was the alignment of organizational purpose and physician involvement in that mission. While we had many excellent physicians who practiced in the hospital, there was only a limited physician formation process that engaged them in its mission.

The future goal was to ensure we continued and expanded, where applicable, those things that supported Catholic identity. We needed to institute a process that documented our actions to ensure that future generations would sustain those practices that maintained and reinforced our mission focus. The second was to integrate physician and hospital alignment concerning enhancing the Catholic identity of CHRISTUS St. Michael Health System. Chapter 9 will outline the ministry's intentional actions to move them to be a virtuous organization.

Summary

The chapter has discussed how Catholic health care has evolved over the years and continues to express and desire to remain faithful to its founders' legacy. The history of the Sisters of Charity of the Incarnate Word and the ministry they established in Texarkana is used as an example of the story of Catholic health care. The role of women (and some men) with religious vocations in creating a legacy for faith-based health care is now changing with the reduction in the number visible in ministries. The need for formation to prepare lay people to assume leadership roles within Catholic (all faith-based) health care is essential. To be successful in the formation process requires that organizations undertake formal and systematic discernment processes. The Catholic Identity Matrix is one example of a tool that focuses clearly on Catholic health care principles. It offers a method to evaluate the organization's practices as measured against the principles and the organization's expressed values. It also provides a process for implementing a plan to improve the areas of need and reinforce strength areas.

Suggested Reading

Catholic Identity or Identities? The book, written by Fr. Gerald Arbuckle, challenges leaders to ground their ministries in Jesus' gospel narrative.

Caritas in Communion: Theological Foundations of Catholic Health Care, by Mother Therese Lysaught, was initially commissioned as a "White Paper" by the Catholic Health Association of the United States. It addresses the issues facing Catholic health care ministries in a time of rapid change. It deals with retaining a Catholic identity in light of the pressure to form cooperative relationships with for-profit entities.

100 Years of Healing, Our History of Healing is a commemorative book compiled by Francine Francis, Director, and Stacye Magness, Coordinator of Marketing/Communications for CHRISTUS St. Michael Health System. The book is available by request and provides a comprehensive history of the ministry (christusstmichael.org/100years).

Chapter Nine

Catholic Identity "Hardwired"

At CHRISTUS St. Michael Health System, our mission is to
*"**extend the healing ministry of Jesus Christ**"*
*by **providing quality, compassionate care** to all.*
(CHRISTUS Health mission statement)

Emily Trancik and Rachelle Barina wrote an article for *U.S. Catholic* in 2015 that posed a challenging question, "What makes a hospital Catholic?"[1] They rightly identify that many Catholic identities are predicated upon external markers such as religious symbols and pictures displayed throughout the property. Others look to the founder's commitment to justice and charity. Finally, some see the practices concerning abortion, euthanasia, and contraception as indicators of the organization's "Catholicity." They correctly identify that "at the heart of the Catholic identity of health care organizations is a belief in God's love and the

---

[1] Emily Trancik, Rachelle Barina, "What Makes a Catholic Hospital Catholic?" *U.S. Catholic Magazine*, March 2015, http://www.uscatholic.org/articles/201503/what-makes-catholic-hospital-catholic-29861.

meaning of Jesus' healing ministry."[2] For an organization to be faithful to its conviction, a mission-driven identity is to internalize the belief in God's love and mercy as expressed through the experience of Christ's teachings and actions.

The Christian faith is generally associated with belief in specific creeds, acceptance of approved dogmas, adherence to a moral code, private morality, involvement with a church community, and a personal relationship to Christ. Jesus' teaching tells us that, in addition, we must practice the faith in our actions. The practice of our faith is manifest in the corporal works of mercy. Jesus tells us in Matthew 25:35-40:

> *For I was hungry, and you gave me food, I was thirsty, and you gave me drink, a stranger, and you welcomed me, naked, and you clothed me, ill, and you cared for me, in prison, and you visited me.' Then the righteous will answer him and say, 'LORD, when did we see you hungry and feed you, or thirsty and give you drink? When did we see you a stranger and welcome you, or naked and clothe you? When did we see you ill or in prison, and visit you? And the king will say to them in reply, 'Amen, I say to you, whatever you did for one of these least brothers of mine, you did for me.'*

---

[2] Ibid.

The command to physically be present to those bodily and materially in need is a concrete requirement. It is a real and often daunting task that means what it says; we must reach out to the poor, the marginalized, those people with physical challenges. Of course, we do not neglect people's spiritual needs, but it is the essential role of Catholic health care to be a prime mover in the corporal works of mercy.

Organizations often have a mission statement that talks about respect for the individual, concern for employees, and a commitment to quality. Faith-based organizations add wording like "demonstrate the love of Christ by providing high-quality care" or some variation of the CHRISTUS mission statement "to extend the healing ministry of Jesus Christ." These statements are often sincere expressions of how the organizations hope to be viewed with their accompanying expression of values.

The ability to maintain a tax-exempt status or to be attractive to a particular group can depend on being seen as a charitable organization. In some instances, this veneer serves as a cover for the organization's real goals concerning market share and profitability. I vividly recall being in a meeting of executives in a for-profit health care company in which the CEO asked each of us the following question: "What is the purpose of our company?" After several people gave statements that seemed like speeches concerning dignity, respect, and quality, one person stood up and said: "To make a profit." The CEO proclaimed with some amusement that the last answer was the most honest of the entire group. I fear that, too often, vertical and horizontal growth, market share, and profitability are the overriding issues addressed in the executive suite of even faith-based organizations.

It has been said that organizations ultimately serve the purpose of perpetuating themselves. That often means the stated mission is the "beard that hides the organization's actual goals." Some Catholic health care has been accused of placing financial return as the organization's principal goal, using the justification that "without a margin, there can be no mission." While there is truth in that statement, it is only a partial truth. Of course, organizations must display good stewardship as part of their responsibility to the mission. Nevertheless, I am convinced that mission and margin are not in tension. Instead, by operating with an individual and organizational focus on the cardinal and theological virtues, we can serve the stated mission and create a community in which individuals can flourish. This environment allows people to have the freedom to "live as well as they can, for as long as they can."

CHRISTUS St. Michael, as an example, uses practices that emphasize virtues and focuses on the fundamental principles of Catholic health care. By their practices, they have moved the community closer to the goal of being one that empowers its residents to make free, informed choices concerning their health care. I will offer examples of how the organization serves its mission by referencing each of the Principles of Catholic health care defined in the CIM. Those principles include solidarity with those who live in poverty, holistic care, respect for human life, participatory community of work and mutual respect, stewardship, and acting in communion with the Church. Each of these principles is evaluated in terms of how well it is integrated into its operation. Appendix B provides a comprehensive listing of the activities that CHRISTUS St. Michael engaged in the Fiscal Year 2016, which was the last year I was the Mission Leader in the system. I have chosen to use only one example of each principle to demonstrate how integration was accomplished.

The first principle I will discuss is solidarity with those living in poverty, and one way it was addressed. The example I will use is CHRISTUS St. Michael's adoption of the HealthConnect Program of premium support initiated under Donna Katen-Bahensky, President and CEO of the University of Wisconsin Hospital and Clinics, in cooperation with the United Way of Dane County, Wisconsin. The University donated $2 million to assist persons with incomes of between 100% and 138% of the poverty guidelines in paying the premium's enrollee portion under the Patient Protection and Affordable Care Act (ACA). I had learned of this program while I was working for a previous employer. Sandy Erickson, Coordinator of the Program for the United Way, and Donna Katen-Bahensky were extremely generous in providing information about how the program was operated. Their assistance was essential in my effort to explain the program to CHRISTUS St. Michael's leadership and gain approval at the corporate level of CHRISTUS Health.

There are substantial differences in the demographics between Madison and Texarkana. Madison is a university/state capital and generally considered a progressive or liberal political environment. Texarkana is predominately light industry, with a significant federal presence with the Red River Army Depot and an agricultural center. Politically, it is part of the conservative area of Northeast Texas. Madison has nearly twice as many people with college degrees (58% to 31%) and a median family income of $62,900 (2018 data) compared to Texarkana's $57,000. Madison is less racially diverse, with 78.4% White, 6.8% Black, and 6.9% Latino or Hispanic. Texarkana is 56% White, 37% Black, and 7.2% Latino or Hispanic. As noted, Madison is a State Capital where Texarkana lies on the border of Arkansas and Texas near the border of two other states, Louisiana and Oklahoma.

Wisconsin had a history of expanding Medicaid coverage with its "Badger Care" program. Texas was one of thirteen states that did not adopt the provisions for Medicaid expansion allowed under the ACA. Texarkana residents who lived on the Arkansas side had access to an expanded health insurance program not available to Texas residents.

Our ministry evaluated the program we had learned about in Madison to help our Texas side residents gain health insurance access. It must be noted that Arkansas did not have an established Medicaid managed care system. There were doubts about whether the State Medicaid or private insurers could "gear-up" for many new enrollees under ACA. The State chose to expand coverage via private plans (Private Option), leveraging private insurance markets, arguing that Arkansas would promote a more efficient system for insuring new enrollees with better access to high-quality providers. A multi-year study supported by The Commonwealth Fund evaluated low-income adults' experiences in Arkansas compared with their Texas counterparts. A summary shows that:

> Arkansas's private option improved access to primary care and prescription medications, reduced reliance on the emergency department, increased use of preventive care, and improved perceptions of quality and health among low-income adults in the state, compared to Texas.[3]

---

[3] Bethany Maylone and Benjamin D. Sommers, "Evidence from the Private Option: The Arkansas Experience," *Commonwealth Fund* (Feb. 22, 2017) https://commonwealthfund.org/publications/issue-briefs/2017/feb/evidence-private-option-arkansas-experience.

The results demonstrated that by access to health insurance coverage, there was an opportunity to substantially improve people's likelihood of having medical homes. Experience has shown that people who have a medical home are much less likely to use emergency rooms for primary care and can have chronic conditions managed more effectively. In addition, preventive services such as immunizations and regular health evaluations are consistently completed. Data we had gathered indicated that people without health insurance showed more often in our emergency room for services routinely offered by primary care. Moreover, patients with chronic conditions often presented advanced symptoms due to avoidance of care because of concern for the expense.

With some modifications, CHRISTUS St. Michael implemented a program similar to the one in Madison to help Texas residents who qualified for the exchange but had such low incomes they could not afford even the most basic policies. The program was aimed at people with incomes between 100% and 150% of the Federal Poverty Guidelines. This group was chosen since they were the most likely to enroll and then either never pay or discontinue paying due to their low income. Enrollees also qualified for cost-sharing reductions through the law, which added actuarial value to the product by paying a larger portion of the overall bill. While it did not solve the problem for those not meeting Medicaid eligibility, it ensured that people at the lowest income levels eligible for Qualified Health Plans offered through the federal marketplace can afford to maintain coverage.

The premium support program was implemented in 2015 and expanded to other CHRISTUS Ministries. The Biden administration continues to support the ACA. The long–term future of the ACA appears to be reliable based on recent court decisions. The program has continued even with CHRISTUS St. Michael's leadership changes because it has become part of how the organization defines "solidarity with the poor." The final part of the story is critical since it demonstrates how intentional action becomes integrated within an organization.

Under federal regulations, CHRISTUS St. Michael could not directly or indirectly control or influence how any money available for the program could be used except for a provision that it must go to eligible applicants. That is, we could not suggest or recommend insurance products for which we were preferred providers or where we had agreements with physicians and other providers aligned with our organization. As was Madison's example, we had to find a not-for-profit, non-aligned, or affiliated organization with the infrastructure to administer the program. It took many months, dozens of phone calls, many meetings, and many no's before we were able to find not merely a suitable candidate but an organization whose mission was to underserved populations.

It was a chance meeting with representatives of the Ark-Tex Council of Governments (ATCOG) concerning improving transportation services for the elderly in the community that revealed the opportunity. ATCOG is a not-for-profit, voluntary association of local governments whose purpose is to promote intergovernmental cooperation. As part of their role, they serve as administer for several state and federal grants for programs for the aging.

We introduced the idea to the agency representatives, who then obtained enthusiastic approval from the agency Executive Director, Chris Brown, to pursue developing the program. This endorsement was a courageous act on Mr. Brown's part as he was newly appointed to the position. He was committing to a program many could see supporting "ObamaCare" in an area considered the "reddest of red" in Texas. It took several months to arrive at a donor agreement that was both compliant with the law's letter and intent. We made what we considered to be an improvement on the application for enrollment in what was now named the "Premium Assistance Program" to assure that people enrolled were eligible and payment to the insurance companies was guaranteed. There was also training necessary for enrollment specialists to ensure that applicants could navigate the process successfully.

These were all technical issues that had to be resolved to the satisfaction of CHRISTUS Health, CHRISTUS St. Michael's community board, and ATCOG. All had to be clear that any funds allocated by CHRISTUS St. Michael could only go for the defined purpose. As donors, we had no direct or indirect control or influence over who would be deemed eligible or receive assistance. CHRISTUS St. Michael only knew the number of enrollees and no other personally identifying information. There was only one last step to making the program operational.

The ATCOG representatives of the ten counties in Texas and Miller County in Arkansas had to give the final approval to implement the program. While this might appear to be a "slam dunk," the fact is that most of the counties would see little effect since they were smaller and more rural than Bowie County, Texas. Also, all the representatives were either Republican or aligned with the Republican party. Finally, the meeting to which I was invited to outline the program was also attended by representatives of Senator Ted Cruz. I was somewhat apprehensive of gaining approval for what many would consider an "ObamaCare" program. After my brief presentation, there was a robust discussion around the issues presented. During what I would term a productive conversation, one of Senator Cruz's representatives stated, "This is just what the Senator is looking for, communities to take responsibility for their residents' well-being."

It was abundantly clear that the county representatives acknowledged CHRISTUS St. Michael's involvement and legacy of concern for the well-being of the communities it serves. The recognition was that this was not a self-serving act but an expression of faithfulness to our mission statement that allowed this group to look beyond partisan considerations. The project also invited ATCOG to be part of the mission to improve the overall community well-being. Since the program's introduction, hundreds of individuals and families have been assisted to gain health insurance. The prudence, courage, and just actions of CHRISTUS St. Michael and ATCOG made this result possible. It is a demonstration of the charity (love) that allows God's kingdom to be expressed in this action.

The second principle identified by the CIM is holistic care. The creators of the CIM define holistic care:

Holistic care is the healing of the whole person, in and through caring relationships. Each person is an inseparable unity of body and spirit (1 Cor 15:44). Catholic health care institution seeks to care for the whole person in an integrated, compassionate manner, attending to the physical, psychological, relational, and spiritual dimensions of each patient's existence.[4]

---

[4] Ascension Health and Veritas Institute of the University of St. Thomas, *The Catholic Identity Matrix: General Information*, (St. Paul, MN: Veritas Institute, 2020), 6.

This explanation is clear and unambiguous. Several types of practitioners claim to be holistic when advocating alternative diets or naturally occurring remedies for preventing or dealing with illness. Holistic care from CHRISTUS St. Michael's perspective requires that the person's physical, emotional, spiritual, and current social situation all be considered in the "care plan." It takes a coordinated team of caregivers to ensure that the care plan includes holistic interventions (processes to improve patient functioning). I will use CHRISTUS St. Michael's Palliative care program as my example to demonstrate their deliberate action concerning holistic care.

A general discussion of the efficacy of Palliative care has taken place. I wish to describe how Palliative care matured from a complementary, infrequently requested service by physicians practicing in the CHRISTUS St. Michael Health Center to one in which a request for a consultation has become a routine practice for persons diagnosed with a life-limiting condition.

Historically, palliative care services within the health center consisted of having a nurse contracted from a local hospice provider see patients with chronic pain issues. The nurse worked under the supervision of a Board-Certified palliative care physician who also had a contractual relationship with the hospice company. The service was involved with approximately 250 patients per year, or less than 2% of all adult admissions. By comparison, the enhanced program subsequently initiated 1481 adult patients in the fiscal year 2019 or 13% of all adult admissions. The improvement resulted from a values-based decision-making process undertaken to identify opportunities for improving the service suggested by the CIM survey.

It was concluded that there were several barriers to effectiveness as we evaluated the service's performance in relation to our mission. First, having the service as an outside contract with a hospice provider created a misunderstanding of the two distinct care types (hospice and palliative). Second, because of this "blurring of the lines," the patients seen were often far advanced in their illness. Third, the physicians did not identify the service as a priority due to the limited commitment of resources invested in the service. Finally, in some instances, particularly with oncology patients, the palliative service was seen as competing instead of complementing the Oncology care plan.

Coinciding with the evaluation we began as part of our commitment to address the opportunities for improvement identified in the CIM was the planned retirement of the contracted nurse and the relocation of the Palliative care physician. A coordinated effort between the departments responsible for Case Management, Mission Integration, and Finance developed a palliative care program plan built upon the outline suggested by the Center to Advance Palliative Care (CAPC). As members of that organization, we could use resources and visit other group members to share ideas. Management's decision created a palliative care program consistent with our aim to provide holistic care to patients with a life-limiting illness.

The program was designed to coordinate with primary care providers who already serve referred patients and find medical homes for those in need. Early identification of patients who could benefit from palliative consultation was deemed to be critical. Education and communication with hospitalists (physicians who specialize in serving inpatient populations) began. A palliative care nurse was assigned to work in the emergency room shortly after implementing the program to improve the ability to identify patients who could benefit at the earliest possible point. It was also determined that maintaining documentation that compared our performance against "benchmarked" data was essential to evaluate the performance and confirm it was addressing our desire to provide holistic care to the identified patient population.

The proposed program required a substantial investment in system resources. That commitment of support also demonstrated the organization's dedication to providing holistic care to the identified patients. It also required a considerable effort to recruit and train the staff to provide the quality outcome service we envisioned. Fortunately, the program was able to retain the services of an Advanced Practice Nurse certified in palliative care to support us in training and assisting the staff. Staffing consists of three registered nurses, an Advance Practice Nurse, a social worker, and two clinical pharmacists assigned to provide 10 hours of consultation per week. A specific chaplain was assigned from the Spiritual Care Department to consult with each palliative patient and participate in team care planning meetings. There is a physician to supervise the program who devotes 20 hours per month to that duty.

It was postulated that an effort to introduce palliative care early after diagnosing a life-limiting illness produces the best results. To test that hypothesis required that the program measure many variables against benchmark standards or compared with patients receiving no interventions. The palliative care team produces a written report monthly to the Palliative Care Committee made up of physicians, nursing, administration, finance, mission integration, and community board members. It compares such data as admissions avoided, the volume of patients in which a consult was ordered, assessment of pain, advance care plans discussed and completed, the functional capacity of the patient at the time of assessment, and length of stay against Palliative Care Quality Network (PCQN) data. CHRISTUS St. Michael has seen more patients earlier in the illness progression, as evidenced by higher functional performance scores. They have also been able to reduce the length of stay as an inpatient and in the ICU. Weaning from ventilators is accomplished in a shorter time, avoiding many of the complications attendant with ventilators.

The data support the program's efficacy. Patient/family satisfaction scores demonstrate the benefit of the chaplain and social worker's involvement in dealing with the patient and family's life situation and their psychological and spiritual needs. The fact is that family meetings that include the chaplain and social worker are twice as frequent as comparable palliative care programs. The chaplain's services are not documented in the report since PCQN provides no comparable data. Data to support and improve the provision of Spiritual Care services is maintained. I would be hopeful that national benchmarks, using information such as CHRISTUS St. Michael, can be developed to reflect the impact of Spiritual Care services more accurately.

The expanded Palliative Care Program was initiated because it improved holistic care provided to patients and families in the most critical need of such "wrap-around" care. The program was directed to document that it could meet that expectation by reducing readmissions for inpatient hospitalization. As a matter of good stewardship, the program was challenged to be able to demonstrate cost avoidance. Because reimbursement for palliative services, which mainly focus on early intervention, is unpredictable, the program was not burdened with unrealistic revenue projections. CHRISTUS St. Michael shows its commitment to this program and the concept of holistic care through its commitment to resources. The Vice President of Finance, Glen Boles, is firmly committed to its mission and values.

He is one of the few financial leaders I have known who can feel comfortable making rounds in the clinical areas and defines the organization as a "ministry." Chris Karam and his successor, Jason Rounds, as presidents, demonstrated their commitment by approval of the allocation of resources. That support extends to the managers and associates who provide the service. Jason Adams, who was appointed President in February 2021, has pledged to continue the commitment as part of the "mission of extending the healing ministry of Jesus Christ."

The Palliative Care Program allows the patient and family to have hope that results from being cared for with love. Moreover, it allows all patients, family, and caregivers to make well-informed and prudent decisions. By implementing the palliative service, the organization showed intentionality in its commitment to act on behalf of those for whom care was provided.

The third principle, respect for human life, is often thought of as the most controversial due to the political/ethical issues surrounding a "women's right to choose." I will present an example of how CHRISTUS St. Michael has reframed the issue to show how, by providing a service consistent with Catholic health care's mission and values, that freedom to make an autonomous decision is made available. People's ability to make autonomous and well-reasoned decisions is a fundamental right if an organization is intentional in the commitment to respect for human life.

As noted previously, part of the ability to make informed health care decisions is based on access to health care professionals.

Chris Karam, whom I have mentioned frequently within this work, was a steadfast advocate for the idea that each person should have access to a medical home. The Primary Care Collaboration defines "the medical home as a model of primary care that is patient-centered, comprehensive, team-based, coordinated, accessible, and focused on quality and safety.[5] Medical homes' availability for those with limited coverage insurance (high co-pays and deductibles) or often no health insurance created a barrier to access.

Too often, primary care is provided in the emergency room. There is the perception that care in that setting is mandatory irrespective of the ability to pay. That perspective is only partially correct. The Emergency Medical Treatment and Active Labor Act (EMTALA), also termed the "antidumping law," was enacted in 1986 to ensure that care was provided to individuals experiencing emergency medical conditions (EMC).

An emergency medical condition is defined as "a medical condition manifesting to itself by acute symptoms of sufficient severity (including severe pain) such that the ab-

---

[5] "Defining the Medical Home," *Patient-Centered Primary Care Collaborative* (Primary Care Collaborative, January 17, 2019), https://www.pcpcc.org/about/medical-home.

sence of immediate medical attention could reasonably be expected to result in -- (i) placing the health of the individual in serious jeopardy, (ii) serious impairment to bodily functions, or (iii) serious dysfunction of any bodily organ or part." (Kauffman v. Franz, 2009 U.S. Dist. LEXIS 88749 (E.D. Pa. Sept. 24, 2009)[6]

The law requires that each person presenting to a Medicare-participating emergency room be given a Medical Screening Examination (MSE). Nevertheless, EMTALA intentionally omitted a hospital requirement to provide uncompensated stabilizing treatment for individuals with medical conditions determined not to be an EMC. Therefore, such individuals are not eligible for further uncompensated examination and treatment beyond the MSE. It was believed that this restriction would limit the number of non-emergent cases that would present at ERs. It did not achieve this goal.

The main reason the goal was unattainable was the difficulty for a patient with Medicaid or no insurance to get an appointment with the community's limited number of primary care providers. CHRISTUS St. Michael, along with the University of Arkansas School of Medicine, created the

---

[6] US Legal, "Find a Legal Form in Minutes," *Emergency Medical Condition Law and Legal Definition*, USLegal, Inc., accessed January 20, 2021, https://definitions.uslegal.com/e/emergency-medical-condition/

Texarkana Community Clinic and its companion pediatric service "All for Kids" in 2009 to address the critical issue of access to care for those with limited resources. CHRISTUS St. Michael financially supported the program but recognized that it was limited in terms of the resources needed to address the problem adequately. Therefore, it was determined that having a health care provider designated as a Federally Qualified Health Center was a desirable goal.

The effort to secure funding for a new FQHC was not successful because the federal government had limited new centers' creation. The alternative was to seek to persuade an existing FQHC to locate an office in Texarkana. It was determined that a Texas location would be the most useful. The decision to locate in Texas required that we find a provider with a Texas license to operate.

It was decided that the East Texas Border Health FQHC, located in Marshall and Longview, Texas, was available. Unfortunately, at that time, the center was not in a financial position to expand. Moreover, the evidence was that the center's services range would not adequately address Texarkana's need. After much deliberation and negotiation between the parties, a decision to expand the center's activity into Texarkana was accomplished. The expansion required a substantial commitment of financial resources and professional consultation on CHRISTUS St. Michael. The organization's governing board was reorganized to allow for diverse community input and health care professional expertise. The organization was renamed Genesis PrimeCare to reflect its enhanced commitment to respect for life and the role the organization planned in empowering people to flourish. Finally, an administrative team with broader health care experience was recruited to improve the business operation's performance. The transition from the Texarkana Community Clinic to Genesis PrimeCare began in December 2012. It was a full two years before the administrative and clinical improvements would be fully realized.

Since Genesis PrimeCare became fully operational in 2015 it has had a significant impact on the community's access to primary care services. The number of visits affirms that assertion. Specifically, there has been an increase from 24,663 patient visits in one Texas location in 2015 to 64,073 patient visits in 2019.[7] Services have been extended to a conveniently located Arkansas location as well. Through an active effort to coordinate care with CHRISTUS St. Michael, there has been a considerable increase in the number of people who now have a medical home. The range of services offered includes mental health, dental, pediatrics, dermatological, pharmacy, obstetrics/

---

[7] The number of patient visits at the Genesis PrimeCare clinics in Texas and later in Arkansas (2016) was used with permission from East Texas Border Health's administration. The legal entity is operating as Genesis PrimeCare.

gynecological, and primary care services. I will highlight one service that is a coordinated effort between Genesis PrimeCare and CHRISTUS St. Michael to demonstrate respect for life and determination to allow patients freedom of choice.

Until 2015 the obstetric/gynecological services of Genesis PrimeCare were limited. Moreover, the need for prenatal care for expectant, low-income mothers was restricted. "Medicaid mothers" were not able to be seen by Dr. Johnny Jones, the physician treating the substantial portion of the "at-risk" population until they were no longer in the "Medicaid Pending" status. This limitation was a result of a stipulation in the physician's contract with another provider. The situation was unacceptable to Dr. Jones since prenatal care for these mothers was essential in his professional opinion. Waiting for the Medicaid status to clear could take precious days and even weeks before the woman could be seen.

The association with Genesis PrimeCare offered Dr. Jones the opportunity to see patients even during the period when their Medicaid status was pending. Dr. Jones was not negotiating for money or other material gains; his concern was the ability to serve his patients, many experiencing "high-risk" pregnancies. He desired to work with the mothers, their support groups, and community resources to ensure that the mother and child's well-being was maintained. By working within the medical home model, mother, baby, and support group could be offered the prospect of good health for all concerned and the chance to flourish. The decision was no longer a binary choice (have or not have), but one in which the opportunity to thrive could be realistically offered. In 2019, Dr. Jones delivered 433 babies considered to be at high risk. During his tenure with Genesis PrimeCare, he has delivered more than 1,700 babies. These were children born to families that were given an option due to the efforts of CHRISTUS St. Michael and Genesis PrimeCare's commitment to the dignity of each person and the respect for life.

The decision to partner with an FQHC that required an "organizational overhaul" was an act of courage and faith, faith in the sense that it was an intentional effort to practice the Christian principle expressed in the mission statement. It was an act of justice to assure access to care for vulnerable populations was available. Moreover, it provided an opportunity to assist those in need to have a reasonable alternative to abortion.

The fourth principle to examine is a participatory community of work and mutual respect. The CIM information guide defines this principle as:

> The associate (employee) is the primary stakeholder for this principle. Made in God's image, people can develop authentically only if they are allowed to use their God-given intelligence and freedom to achieve shared goals

and to build and sustain right relationships with one another.[8]

Before you can build relationships based on mutual trust, you need to take an honest look at your motivations for adopting a participatory workplace approach. Often, there is an imbalance of power between the health care organization (as the party that holds access to crucial resources) and the affected population (patients and bedside caregivers). The use of terminology such as "frequent flyers" implies a certain degree of condescension or hierarchy, a barrier to caring between caregivers and patients. Furthermore, the situations in which organizations work and operating methods they employ often create distance between associates, which does not help build relationships based on mutual respect and trust.

Sponsoring a participatory workplace is an intentional act. An organization's obligation, such as a ministry, is caring for people, "with the more able and the less able serving each other."[9] The responsibility of caring has moved from the family to large and often impersonal organizations that may be viewed with suspicion and a lack of trust. To over-

---

[8] Ascension, 7.

[9] Robert K Greenleaf, *Servant Leadership: A Journey into the Nature of Legitimate Power and Greatness*, ed. Larry C. Spears (Mahwah, NJ: Paulist Press, 2002), 62.

come these trust barriers, an organization must be courageous enough to ask questions like: Are we taking this position to improve how we are perceived in the community or targeting particular groups to gain favor? Is the purpose primarily to reduce costs or use outsourcing to reduce costs with no measurable change in quality? Is it because a donor asked for a paragraph on participation in their pledge? Is it because your organization believes that participation can considerably improve the short- and longer-term impact of association satisfaction? Is the practice to facilitate associate identification with the ministry's goals? Importantly, is it because your organization recognizes that associates are not passive recipients of aid but persons of dignity responsible for their future skills and aspirations?

Once the commitment to a participatory workplace is made, the means of implementation is critical. Questions such as, "With whom should my organization work become vital?" The use of consulting services was central at CHRISTUS St. Michael when the corporate office directed each ministry to use a particular organization to arrive at appropriate staffing levels for each location. The group used an algorithm as the basis for establishing staffing models. Those models did not adequately address the operational situations encountered in Texarkana. As a result, there was an undermining of a sense of participation on the part of managers. The process revealed a need to assure that associates are suitably represented without controlling their leadership or spokesperson selection. Basing such critical decisions as staffing on a computer model seemed to offer an effective method for dealing with this vexing issue. The actual result was an undermining of the idea foundational to a participatory workgroup. The key idea is that people can genuinely mature only if they can use their God-gifted intelligence and freedom to achieve shared goals and build and sustain the right relationships. As a result of utilizing a Values-Based Decision-Making Process (VBDMP), CSMHS, in cooperation with the consulting group, effectively implemented a program to improve staffing.

Common ways of describing an organization's relation to associates are to refer to them as a key or the most critical asset. While unintended, this description of associates is a way of objectifying and depersonalizing the people who make up your organization. Objectification of individuals reduces them to replacement parts, tools that serve a particular function without an appreciation for and recognition of the unique experiences, skills, and cultural knowledge they bring to the workplace? Moreover, it denies ownership of the mission as being part of the common good. A participatory workplace is founded on the idea that people thrive in relationships with others. We are nurtured through our relations with others, including the organizations in which we earn a living.

By preventing associates from opportunities to use their skills to embrace the organization's mission, we are also blocking efforts to achieve the two principal purposes of maintaining a participatory workplace. The CIM document describes those purposes as:

> First, an organization serves the "external" human good of the wider community when it produces goods or services that meet authentic human needs, when it operates responsibly in its relationships with stakeholders, and when it provides employment that allows people to enjoy a decent standard of living. Second, the organization promotes its "internal" common good when it fosters the emergence of a community among its associates, i.e. when it enables associates to grow as persons through their relations with others in the task of serving the "external" common good.[10]

Respect for each associate's dignity is reflected in how we structure safe working conditions, providing a fair wage and benefits program. It includes the opportunity for advanced education as well as growth in responsibility. The organization should have an active and ongoing program of continuing education, not merely technical skills training. There should be an ongoing effort to assure that associates are engaged, at the appropriate level, to ensure involvement

---

[10] Ascension, 6.

in developing the organization's strategic plan concerning the ministry's mission.

For associates to be fully engaged required two critical assumptions to be considered. First, there had to be a fundamental belief in the principle of subsidiarity. Decisions ought to be handled by the competent unit closest to the action. Authority over one's work should be allowed to be made, as often as possible, by those who are directly affected. Subsidiarity involves those with more formal authority to act as support for the frontline workers. The idea of "servant leadership" is fundamental within an organization that endeavors to have the more participatory engagement of associates called under the subsidiarity principle.

Servant leadership has become a popular style, thanks to the writing of Robert Greenleaf. In this model, the leader serves as a servant. The leader's task is to make the space for those being served to become stronger, informed, spontaneous, and autonomous. Is the organization one that empowers people to become servant leaders? My friend, John Bussen, taught me that the mark of a good servant leader was in answer to the question, "Were the people around the leader permitted to be free?" Being free meant being able to pursue that which was good for the individual and the organization. Greenleaf writes that the test of a servant leader is:

Do those served grow as persons? Do they, while being served, become healthier, wiser, freer, more autonomous, more like themselves to become servants? And, what is the effect on the least privileged in society? Will they benefit or a least not be deprived further.[11]

Both Bussen and Greenleaf are making the point that being a servant leader starts with a desire to serve others. Servant leadership was built on this foundation of commitment to individual action and social justice. Thus, servant leadership's concept aligns with the idea expressed in this book concerning living a virtuous life as both an individual decision and collective action. The highest priority is to seek that which is good and is best expressed through acting in line with the cardinal and theological virtues discussed throughout this work. Doing the right things can lead to performance improvement, but doing the right thing using the principles embedded in the cardinal and theological virtues allows for God's will to be done. It means leading with the view toward being faithful to the mission statement through being intentional in our actions and service decisions. It is an act of prudence in undertaking intentional actions directed at supporting those who serve the organization.

---

[11] Greenleaf, 27.

The second critical assumption was that for a person to make a free decision (seeking the good), he or she must also be informed. Like other faith-based organizations, CHRISTUS St. Michael uses a method termed Values-Based Decision-Making Process (VBDMP) to discern the proper course of action the organization should undertake. When issues that directly impact the ability to be faithful to the organization's values and mission are called into question, the process is used. VBDMP involves the practice of discernment to arrive at decisions consistent with how the mission is carried forward. Earlier, I used Panicola and other authors to describe discernment as not merely an intellectual exercise. Instead, the authors describe discernment as "the skill or virtue of perceiving and distinguishing degrees of value between diverse factors when making decisions."[12] Discernment includes the virtue of prudence but is not exclusively a product of reason. The authors point out that discernment includes a spiritual component involving introspection and contemplating one's thoughts, desires, and conduct combined with the ability to reason as essential in arriving at informed decisions that allow the person to flourish.

VBDMP includes a broader base than is available merely through reason. To prepare associates to participate in the decision-making process in a manner consistent with

---

[12] Panicola, et al., 65.

the principle of subsidiarity required a commitment to an ongoing education and formation process. VBDMP requires technical knowledge for both clinical and business questions. It also involves an understanding of Catholic health care principles, awareness of the founders' legacy, and an appreciation of the process of contemplation.

In 2008, the organization worked with CHRISTUS Health's corporate resources to create a program to address these decision-making elements. It was initially anticipated to be an 18-month, structured process to align goals, behaviors, and processes to consistently achieve excellence in each of four directions—clinical quality, service quality, business literacy, and community value. The original intent would appear to be consistent with what one could see in a leadership development educational process for almost any organization. Fidelity to the mission and identification as a ministry could be seen as implied within the community value direction. The original program did not demonstrate the intentional obligation for fidelity to its mission and values. The format to deal with what were identified as opportunities for improvement was off-site structured learning workshops to develop leaders' skills "to enable the achievement of organizational goals, as well as to improve individual leadership performance and organizational consistency."[13] They were named Leadership Development Institutes (LDI) that relied on data-driven information designed to provide participants with the skills and tools needed to implement the organization's goals.

I believe the lack of focus on formation resulted from the fact that there was still a strong representation of religious women providing Spiritual Care (chaplains) services. I have already spoken about the compelling presence that the Sisters of the Incarnate Word embodied. The sisters wore the more traditional habit with a simple wimple. Having nuns, even those not from the sponsoring congregation, gave Catholic hospitals an identity. Although it was important for "lay" administrators to appreciate the Catholic identity, there was far less pressure to act as a spokesperson or develop a relationship with the local bishop. The perception was that the Sister's main concern was serving the poor. Running the business was the responsibility of the lay administrator. From my experience, I can state without qualification that nothing could be further from the actual situation. I have previously noted that the sisters who led Catholic health care represented a remarkable group of

---

[13] CHRISTUS, like many other health care organizations, was relying on the Studer Group consultation organization, which is well-known for assisting health care organizations "transform" to meet the need of a complex and ever-changing health care environment.

highly skilled, educated, and focused leaders. The difficulty was that the numbers of religious women (nuns) available to act as CEOs began to diminish. The reduction in religious congregation members in leadership within Catholic health care meant that identifying its formal authentication as a ministry was also lessened.

As sponsors, the sisters were seen as "owning the mission" due to their chosen life. Also, the role of mission leader in organizations had been designed to have a member of the sponsoring congregation be the "moral compass" of the organization when lay leadership became the typical model. By moral compass, they were asked to be the conscience of the organization. The Catholic Church's *Catechism* defines conscience as "a judgment of reason whereby the human person recognizes the moral quality of a concrete act that he is going to perform, is in the process of performing, or has already performed" (*CCC* 1778). Conscience is a "judgment of reason" that determines whether an act is right or wrong. Laypeople were called to fill that role as sisters continued to retire without being replaced from within their congregations, but often without the formal authority given to the nuns.

The loss of sisters visible in the ministry led to a need to focus attention on formation. Formation involved transforming leadership training from purely technical skills to one which recognized the importance of discernment. Catholic health care had always had those with religious vocations to serve as the organization's prophetic voice. Like Sr Carmelita, of whom I spoke earlier, religious leaders were what Greenleaf called "conceptualizers."[14] Conceptual talent sees the big picture, anticipates the unexpected, and effectively uses formal and informal (persuasive) power. The conceptualizers effectively balanced the need to deal with day-to-day operational issues and pursue organizational goals with the broader mission-focused purpose. These leaders from the founding congregations were the moral compass (conscience) and the organization's conceptual and operational leaders.

Now, the "face of the ministry" would have to be lay leaders, some of whom were not Catholic. Even when the leader was Catholic (several systems had to be Catholic as an unwritten qualification for CEOs), the role of visible representative of the Catholic identity was not possible to be fulfilled in the same manner as it was with the sisters. CHRISTUS Health, like many Catholic health care systems, created formation programs for executive leadership. These programs served the purpose of giving executives the foundational information necessary to understand the founders' purpose.

CHRISTUS Health also spent time encouraging developing the skills, which I will repeat since they are critical. Discernment includes a spiritual component involving in-

---

[14] Greenleaf, 79.

trospection, contemplating your thoughts and desires and conduct, combined with reason as essential in arriving at informed decisions that allow the person to flourish. The issue then became one of "cascading" the leaders' experience to those throughout the organization. The servant-leader model entailed empowering others within the organization to help develop the associate's ability to thrive within the workplace. CHRISTUS St. Michael took the original concept behind the initial LDI project, expanding it to include the additional elements that would improve operational performance and deal with virtuous living and understanding what discernment meant within the mission's context and values of the organization.

The practice of the LDI continued beyond the initial 18-month project period and continues even today. It is a process that is "hardwired" into CHRISTUS St. Michael and expanded to every ministry within CHRISTUS Health. Each session is fundamentally directed toward the formation of "front-line" managers. The session has an operational focus to assure adherence and understanding of the current goals of the organization. There is also a substantial effort to invite spiritual growth through reflection and stories from scripture to show the connection between Catholic health care beliefs and actions.

A full section of each session is devoted to inviting a representative of a companion organization (i.e., partner organizations) to reinforce the ministry's interconnectedness within the community. A portion of the meeting is set aside to formalize how to cascade the information to all organization associates to share knowledge and empower others. Finally, there is a section of each LDI in which a manager is invited to give a personal witness concerning their reason for working within Catholic health care. The title given in this section of the meeting is the "passion" story. The stories reveal a good deal about the witness. Moreover, it is an opportunity for all to understand that shared values serve to bring us together. The passion stories are the "proof statement" that the servant-leader and participatory workplace are present and active in its culture.

The fifth CIM principle to be dealt with is stewardship. The CIM information manual describes stewardship as:

A good steward is respectful of all resources placed into his or her care, including financial assets, human talents, and natural resources. Everything we have received is part of our patrimony, and we will be judged on how well and productively we have used it (Mt 25:14-30).[15]

Stewardship has most often been identified in more narrow terms than the CIM description suggests. The principle is generally defined in terms of financial performance

---

[15] Ascension, 6.

and sound financial management. Yet, if the CIM description is accurate, then stewardship involves the appropriate use of gifts we are given. Have the resources been made available to promote the common good, create more access to care, and find ways to be wiser in developing business partnerships? Stewardship requires all those involved to ensure that we are doing the right things for the right reasons. Collaboration is a word that is used very loosely to describe a variety of personal and business relations. Sofield and Juliano identify four levels of what is termed collaboration. They are coexistence, communication, cooperation, and collaboration.[16] Within this work, I have used the word collaborative or collaboration in a precise manner.

The best way to clarify what I mean by the statement above is to describe the various ways the term collaboration is used. I will again use Sofield and Juliano as my reference in describing what they call levels of collaboration. The first level is coexistence, in which individuals or groups share something in common. For instance, I went to high school with 824 others. I have a shared experience with my classmates but are independent of one another. The second level is communication, which is the sharing of information relevant to the parties involved. Problems with communica-

---

[16] Loughlan Sofield and Carroll Juliano, *Collaboration: Uniting Our Gifts in Ministry* (Notre Dame, IN: Ave Maria Press, 2000), 18.

tion are often the cause of disagreement. The fact is that communication may move the parties toward common ground but does not require shared values. The third level is cooperation, in which the parties recognize they do not exist in isolation. The parties recognize the value of working together even though such cooperation may be time or project limited. The final level, true collaboration, as used within this work, involves the groups acknowledging a joint mission, an articulation of that mission with commonly established goals, and a "decision to identify, value and unite the various gifts that each possesses."[17] As I discuss strategic planning efforts and actions taken to support that plan, I use the term collaboration in business and patient care as described in the fourth level.

Around 2014, CHRISTUS Health created a strategic planning process called Compass 2020 that focused on crucial destination points and critical pathways that would lead to excellence in clinical and operational efficiency, commitment to the communities served, and financial performance to sustain the ministries. The original version of the plan's elements began with a "top-box" goal of a specific financial margin (profit percentage) for each ministry in the system. The implied purpose of the goal was to assure the ministries could be sustained.

---

[17] Ibid, 19.

CHRISTUS St. Michael intentionally reframed the top-box to reflect what the intent of the primary goal represented. That is, the goal was restated to reflect the mission commitment to serving our community, increasing access to care, and giving preference for the poor as a result of sustaining a financially viable organization. Financial performance was the appropriate means to the ministry goals; it was not the goal in and of itself. The point being made was that CHRISTUS St. Michael and all the ministries in the CHRISTUS system did not exist to increase the "shareholder" value. Instead, our goal was driven by the elements included in the mission and core values statement that we proclaimed represented our intentions.

The examples of collaborative programs described herein, like Premium Support, show the intentional commitment of resources to assist underserved people without health insurance. The ongoing support, both financial and through involvement on the Board of Trustees, has assured that medical homes are available for low-income residents. Others, such as the "Go Noodle" program that partners with local school districts to promote health literacy among the young, demonstrate service commitment. The Parish Nurse Program sponsored in cooperation with Catholic Charities of the Tyler Diocese serves several churches of various denominations in diverse and urban locations to have better availability of maintenance support for those with chronic illness. CHRISTUS St. Michael was instrumental in providing the space and financing the remodeling of space to create a mental health crisis intervention service. The local community mental health provider operates the service to assist people with acute mental health issues who need a safe place to recover.

One program that demands special attention because it touched so many stewardship elements is a project conducted in collaboration with The Texas Dental Association's Smiles Foundation. The foundation operates the Texas Mission of Mercy (TMOM) outreach program to provide dental services within underserved communities. Dan Ford, then Director of Mission Integration, was aware of the program and arranged to schedule a 2-day clinic in Texarkana. Subsequently, Dan was promoted and transferred to another ministry within CHRISTUS. The co-chair took a position with another organization. The project was left with no formal leadership. It was through the insistence of Chris Karam and the efforts of Sue Johnson, Director of Advocacy and Community Planning, Fred Brantley, Controller, Mary Catherine Haynes (Hospital Board Member), and Milburn Haynes, DDS, that the project was able to be sustained. I was fortunate to join the organization at that point, which gave me a "ring-side" seat to seeing a mission-focused organization operate. Through conversations with TMOM board member Dr. Mike Geisler, I learned of the organization's faith-based purpose in reaching out to the poor, much as in Jesus' ministry. The hospital emergency room experienced approximately 130 primary dental visits per month from people without dental insurance. We could do little for these patients who were suffering from unyielding pain and often severe infections. The TMOM was an effort to deal with the practical issue of inappropriate use of the ER and the desire to express love for our neighbors.

Along with several other dentists, Drs. Haynes and Geisler wanted to assist people experiencing dental problems but unable to access care. CHRISTUS St. Michael and the local dentists had the common concern for access to care for the poor as a way of demonstrating the presence of Jesus through the action of his followers. Both parties agreed to invest the financial resources, time, and talent necessary to accomplish the dual goals of reducing unnecessary use of the ER and showing the mercy of God's love for vulnerable people.

The first clinic was held in 2011 in the gymnasium of Texas High School, with janitorial and security services offered at no charge by the school district. The hospital food, security, and maintenance service vendors all donated their time to assure safety, cleanliness, and food availability for participants. Local restaurants provided food for the volunteers. The school administration and board were entirely "on board" with the method and purpose. Since that time, Texarkana has held more TMOM clinics than any other community in the state of Texas. The clinics have served as an introduction to Genesis PrimeCare's dental services and reduced the use of CHRISTUS St. Michael's emergency room for dental services to a small number. Finally, the clinics provided an opportunity for hundreds of CHRISTUS St. Michael and community members to share their love with a diverse group of people that they likely would never have met otherwise.

The intentional actions for which the TMOM is an example demonstrated how prudence, courage, and justice combine with an active faith, resulting in an expression of charity that could not have been easily duplicated. It offered the opportunity to "do good" as well as actively show regard for others.

Finally, while it is not appropriate to reproduce the strategic plan created by CHRISTUS St. Michael, I can offer some insights from Chris Karam, who was the CEO at the time. These thoughts are reflected in a letter Chris sent to then-President-Elect Trump (see appendix C), which outlines some specific ideas concerning stewardship that he has kindly allowed me to share.

First, Karam identifies pharmaceutical and supply costs as items in which the federal government's involvement through the Medicare and Medicaid programs' buying power could substantially increase competition and reduce cost. Second, he believes, "we need a single billing form for all insurance companies. This action would decrease back-office functions." Third, the use of best practices in the provision of care is critical to reducing costs. CHRISTUS St.

Michael, as well as the entire CHRISTUS Health system, has worked diligently to implement this strategy since it results in better outcomes, allows for better collaboration with the patient (an essential component of treating with dignity), and reduces the length of stay in the most expensive treatment settings. Fourth, Karam advocates high-risk pools for those with chronic conditions or conditions brought on by a catastrophic event. The point being made by Karam is that with some effort, we can transform the health care system. By making changes such as he outlines, we can serve those in need in a way that best utilizes the God-given resources we have available. His message is a direct appeal to the core of how the CIM documents describe Stewardship.

The final principle identified in the CIM is to act as a ministry of the church. This principle is defined as:

A Catholic health care institution holds in sacred trust the healing ministry of Jesus, which it has inherited from both its founders and the larger Church (1Cor 12:4-13). Recognizing that its mission arose from the Church and from an institutional fidelity to the Church's teachings, the institution acts as a ministry of the Catholic Church, observing its ethical and religious directives. It also collaborates with the local Church in the communities.[18]

The Report to the Bishop, referred to within this work, provides ample evidence of the organizations' effort to intentionally act as a church's ministry. A summary of the report shows the effort undertaken to ensure the organization acted according to the principle's intent.

The mission leader ensured that all the organization's policies, procedures, and practices are consistent with the Catholic Church's teachings. Each policy, be it clinical, financial, or quality, has a statement in the Preamble that identifies the principle of Catholic health care, value, or relationship to the mission statement. The mission leader is a member of the administrative team involved with all aspects of the operation. That role includes evaluating relationships with non-Catholic entities for which contractual arrangements, mergers, and acquisitions are being contemplated.

The ministry Spiritual Care Services makes available qualified chaplains at all hours of the day, 7 days per week. Chaplains are assigned to palliative care, surgery, ICU, ER, women's services, the rehabilitation hospital, and medical/surgical services. Additionally, the mission leader is responsible for working with the Director of Spiritual Services to ensure ongoing formation programs are available to all

---

[18] Ascension, 7.

associates. CHRISTUS St. Michael utilizes the Leadership Development Institute for all managers and directors as an ongoing venue for providing spiritual formation experiences. These events are held quarterly. The Mission Leader also holds regular meetings with physicians to discuss the integration of spiritual and physical care.

CHRISTUS St. Michael Board Members are invited to participate in an annual planning retreat. There is a focus on the integration of the mission with the execution of the business plan. The session's focus is planning for a future in which Catholic health care will be severely challenged to maintain focus on Mission while being prudent stewards of the gifts given to us by our Creator.

The organization also has an active Ethics Committee that meets six times per year. The Ethics committee has representation from all aligned physician groups, palliative care, all clinical nursing areas, the CEO, CNE, and CMO. The committee has several subcommittees, namely:

- Patient rights
- Organizational/business ethics
- Advance care planning
- Policy review
- Ethics Consultation Team.

The Ethics Consultation Team is comprised of two certified medical bioethicists. Those individuals are the Chief

Nursing Executive and the Vice President of Mission Integration, who have been provided training through the National Catholic Bioethics Center. Ethics Consultation requests are responded to within 24-hours.

CHRISTUS St. Michael provides over 13% of its operating expense for charity and community benefit. Community benefit includes activities such as physician, nurse, and allied health professional education. Partnership with the FQHC, local school districts, community mental health, homeless services, and the "Spirit of St. Michael" mobile medical clinic is also an essential component. CHRISTUS St. Michael worked in conjunction with Catholic Charities East Texas to establish a Parish Nursing Network in Texarkana. The Health Center also led the community effort to enroll persons in the Health Care Exchange and the Private Option health insurance plans.

CHRISTUS St. Michael provides an Employee Assistance Program (EAP) that provides mental health, chemical dependency, and family assistance. The program also sponsors a health and financial awareness program. The Health Center also provides no-interest loans to associates with short-term acute financial needs. All associates receiving loans are also enrolled in a financial counseling service to assist them in "money management." In addition to the EAP, the Spiritual Care Department has one chaplain assigned to associates to deal with crisis and spiritual assistance times.

CHRISTUS St. Michael is fully committed to each principle of the Catholic Identity Matrix. Its actions demonstrate an intentional attending to what it means to identify as a Catholic health care provider. The organization recognizes that it has been established to provide health care services in the spirit of love and mercy extended first by Jesus and followed through in the founders' actions. CHRISTUS St. Michael also recognizes the need to operate prudently to allow for the ministry's sustainability. Finally, there is a recognition that collaboration with others within the community expands its ability to spread the message of love and mercy fundamental to its mission.

CHRISTUS St. Michael prepared for a CIM survey to occur in March 2020. The Covid-19 pandemic precluded the survey from being conducted. Irrespective, I was involved in reviewing the materials collected to support the ministry's fidelity to Catholic health care principles. I have a high level of confidence that the organization will continue to demonstrate its commitment to its mission when the survey is conducted.

Summary

The executive summary reporting on CHRISTUS St. Michael's Catholic Identity Matrix (CIM) survey prepared by the Veritas Institute states:

These scores are among the highest recorded to date in a CIM application, and are indicative of an institution that has developed the capacity to support the six principles of Catholic health care. In short, CHRISTUS St. Michael has established a comprehensive and capable foundation for systematically advancing its mission as a Catholic health care ministry.[19]

The report identified eight areas where there were opportunities for improvement. CHRISTUS St. Michael has subsequently addressed each of the suggestions. Those improvements include providing a specific written reference to the value or principle addressed in policies and processes. Physician alignment has been improved by integrating CHRISTUS physicians into the Trinity Clinic. The interview process for hiring leaders formally includes questions linked to critical elements of Catholic identity. CHRISTUS St. Michael is now documenting what was previously informal practices to ensure they become "hardwired." Several initiatives directed at support solidarity with the poor have been instituted. Chief among these are the Premium Support program and the creation of the Federally Qualified Health Clinic. Finally, the spiritual care leadership has recruited a more diverse racial, gender, and denominationally affiliated, CPE-trained staff. All of these actions

---

[19] Ibid.

are designed to demonstrate the intentional plan the CHRISTUS St. Michael has "to extend the healing ministry of Jesus Christ."

Suggested Readings

Robert Greenleaf's *Servant Leadership: A Journey into the Nature of Legitimate Power and Greatness* is a must-read for ministry leaders and the governing board members. The book is comprised of essays that give the readers the link between virtue ethics and effective leadership. The book emphasizes service to others. Greenleaf sees organizations' role as creating people who can build a better tomorrow. Servant leadership is well-suited to a mission to provide a community in which people are empowered to flourish.

Food for the Journey: Theological Foundations of the Catholic Healthcare Ministry, written by Juliana Casey, IHM presents the story of Catholic health care as a demonstration of Christ's healing mercy. It provides leaders with insights into the relationship of the health care ministry of the Catholic Church.

Concluding Thoughts

I read a recent article in the *Texarkana Gazette* concerning a Crossing Guard hit by a truck. He was hospitalized in CHRISTUS St. Michael Health System's acute hospital and subsequently in St. Michael Rehabilitation Hospital. The injuries he received were quite severe, requiring 50 days of hospitalization. The story ended with this comment from the patient; "God's house has taken good care of me."[1] The patient's statement is a succinct description of the way I have tried to describe how an institution can be faithful to its mission statement. An institution's ability to fulfill its mission depends on a clear understanding of the elements from which the mission is derived. Within this work, I have made an effort to show the mission statement's why and how to carry it out.

The injured man's statement contains elements of what I have maintained throughout this book. It is both faith and action, individually and corporately, that offers us the opportunity to experience true happiness in life. Despite the challenges experienced by each of us, I have maintained that living a life that embraces the cardinal and theological

---

[1] Karl Richter, "Crossing Guard Hit by Truck in Texarkana to Leave Hospital," *Texarkana Gazette*, November 13, 2020, sec. News.

virtues will allow one to thrive. I have contended that living life in such a manner allows one to make well-informed decisions. Well-informed decision-making for individuals and corporate entities relies on understanding faith that has been handed down through scripture and their interpretation in the Church's teaching. Freedom results from our ability to make appropriate decisions for our situation and are infused with a belief in a Creator God.

I have also declared that there is a corporate responsibility to act in a virtuous manner. This mandate is especially true with regard to the practices of faith-based health care providers. I have singled out Catholic health care because it is the largest provider of such care. Additionally, I have intimate knowledge about Catholic health care organizations' operations both as an outside contractor and an associate within Catholic health care systems.

The organization I have used as a model of what I consider virtuous practices is not perfect. CHRISTUS St. Michael, as well as many other faith-based organizations, have come to realize that it must engage in a continuous effort of discernment to assure they are genuinely carrying on the legacy of the founding religious orders. That is why the Catholic Health Association of the USA (CHA) is leading the effort to assist members in actively evaluating their commitment to such principles as solidarity with the poor, holistic care, respect for life, and subsidiarity. The organizations are called to act as good stewards of the resources that are available to them. Good stewardship allows the ministry to consistently serve the communities within the mission statement's scope and values expressed by the healthcare provider.

The ability of individuals and organizations to act virtuously is becoming more difficult. The Pew Research Center reports that 65% of American adults call themselves Christians when asked about their religion, down from 87% ten years earlier. The religiously unaffiliated are reported to be 26%, up from 17% in 2009.[2] In a post-modern era that can be described as displaying an attitude of cynicism, subjectivism, or relativism, there is a general suspicion of reason and an acute sensitivity to authority's role. This form of thinking denies that there are statements about reality that are objectively true or false. Human beings are not able to know things with certainty. There are no absolute <u>moral</u> values. Dialogues construct reality, knowledge, and value; therefore, they can vary depending on circumstances or the opinion of those affected.

Within this culture of change and conditional values, we are called to embrace the cardinal and theological virtues as individuals and organizations. Indeed, it is counter-

---

[2] "In U.S., Decline of Christianity Continues at Rapid Pace," *Pew Research Center's Religion & Public Life Project*, June 9, 2020, https://www.pewforum.org/2019/10/17/in-u-s-decline-of-christianity-continues-at-rapid-pace/.

cultural in terms of acceptance of moral principles firmly rooted in a belief system that accepts a Creator God who wishes to have a relationship with creation. The individual trends demonstrated by the Pew Research data indicate a movement away from living with confidence in the certainty of God's promises. Post-modern ideas emphasize pleasure and reward as being immediate. It is living for the moment with little to no regard for the consequences of one's actions. It encourages short-term thinking and the quest for immediate gratification. This view of life has a profound impact on how we live personally and act corporately.

I am describing the change in individual behavior regarding religion and our view of values as relative. A change in how we view health care's provision, especially that care provided by faith-based organizations, has changed. The emergence of large-scale government reimbursement with the passage of the Medicare and Medicaid laws in the 1960s and the transition to diagnostic related group (DRG) payment provided an environment that encouraged the profit motive and increased providers' consolidation to promote efficiency. The DRG payment methodology allowed efficient organizations to achieve significant profits by consolidating buying power, establishing standardized (best practices) methods of providing care, and aligning physician practices, emphasizing patient specialties that yielded the highest profit margin.

Many hospitals that began as faith-based terminated their religious affiliations because of the various denomination's desire not to oversee the complex business that health care systems were becoming. Often the name of the hospital retained its denominational identity but operated independently. Within Catholic health care, there was a consolidation of systems in which there would be multiple sponsors rather than a single sponsoring Congregation. This consolidation trend coincided with the reduced availability of nuns to hold the key leadership positions they previously dominated and the need to expand purchasing power, gain access to capital, and increase market influence.

Another major change in organizational structure occurred when many Catholic health care systems became governed under the "Public Juridic Person" model. A public juridic person is a group of laypersons approved by the Roman Catholic Church to oversee and ensure that its health care organization's mission is carried out according to Catholic principles. The principal benefit to the sponsoring congregations who undertook this type of transition is that it allowed the health care system to maintain its Catholic identity and the Sisters to retain reserved powers regarding choosing a system leader and board member approval.

The challenge was and continues to be how organizations designed to maximize market share, efficiency, and profitability align with a Mission Statement that emphasizes a message of ministry. The issue becomes one of defining and then acting upon what is determined to be the end desired. Recently, Catholic health care and other non-profit health care providers have been classified by politicians and some in the public media as just another business entity with a primary goal of generating a profit. The assertion is that profit is the goal instead of the means to the end of "extending the healing presence of Jesus Christ."

The challenge is to assure that the mission is the goal and stewardship of resources is identified as one means to that end. That will require organizations to recruit intentionally and actively provide ongoing formation opportunities to system leaders. It will require the recruitment of persons who demonstrate fidelity to virtuous living and an understanding of what is essential to be faithful to the founder's legacy and the principles of Catholic health care set forth in scripture and Church teaching.

I was recently privileged to assist an effort of the Aquinas Institute of Theology in St. Louis, led by its President, Fr. Mark Wedig, O. P., PhD. and Fr. Michael Mascari, O.P., PhD., Vice President and Academic Dean, to consider ways to address the challenges existing in Catholic health care today. The Aquinas Institute of Theology has trained dozens of mission leaders over more than two decades through its Ashley-O'Rourke Center for Health Ministry. Interviews with many mission leaders within Catholic health care systems revealed that although most systems had programs of formation for leaders, physicians, and front-line associates, there was a need for additional formal education for emerging and existing leaders. The focus would be on giving Catholic and non-Catholic system representatives a firmer understanding of scripture, canon law, the Church's teachings, and leadership principles for mission-driven organizations. The Aquinas Institute of Theology will again be at the forefront by offering a credit-bearing Graduate Certificate in Health Care Mission program to prepare "current and future professionals to foster strategic and collaborative thinking in their organizations so as to ensure faithfulness to their purpose, identity, and values."[3]

It is a commitment to continuing the founders' legacy, encouraging the formation of health care leaders and faithfulness to the cardinal and theological virtues, individually and corporately, that will allow communities to flourish. It is the demonstration of the commitment that CHRISTUS St. Michael, as well as other CHRISTUS locations, have to serve the ministry's mission which makes me even more committed to getting that message out to as many people as possible. CHRISTUS St. Michael is not perfect, but it is as close as it gets in Catholic healthcare.

---

[3] A statement quoted from the Aquinas Institute of Theology's description of the Graduate Certificate in Health Care Ministry's purpose. More information can be obtained at https://www.ai.edu.

Appendix A—Awards and Achievements CHRISTUS St. Michael Health System

Updated March 2020
Used with the permission of CHRISTUS St. Michael Health System

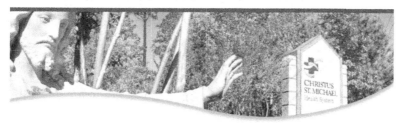

CHRISTUS St. Michael Health System Awards and Achievement

- 50 Tops Cardiovascular Hospitals by IMB Watson Health (2020)
- American College of Cardiology Accreditation-Chest Pain Center with Primary PCI
- IBM Watson Health Top 100 Hospital (2019) with Everest Award (one of only 15 hospitals in the nation to earn)
- Texarkana Gazette Readers' Choice Award Best Hospital (2019)

- Healthcare Financial Management Association MAP Award for High Performance in Revenue Cycle (2019)
- Achievers' 50 Most Engaged Workplaces and Elite 8 Winner in the category of Accountability and Performance
- Healthgrades Awards- Patient Safety Excellence Award (2017, 2018), Outstanding Patient Experience (2017, 2018), Coronary Intervention Excellence Award (2019), Gynecologic Surgery Excellence Award (2018)
- Texas Award for Performance Excellence (all facilities and HH surveyed) (2014)
- Thomson Reuters 100 Top Hospital (2011, 2012)
- AHA/ASA Target: Stroke Honor Roll-Elite– Gold Plus Award Quality Achievement (2017, 2018, 2019)
- Target Stroke Honor Roll – Gold Plus Award (2013, 2014, 2015, 2016)
- Arkansas Department of Health Stroke Care Performance-
- Outstanding Stroke Patient Care (Defect Free Care)- 2016, 2017
- The Joint Commission Accredited
- The Joint Commission Disease-specific certifications - Primary Stroke, Orthopedic Joint Replacement-Hip & Knee, Spine Surgery

- American Diabetes Association Recognized Diabetes Education Program
- Level III Trauma Designation – Arkansas
- Level III Trauma Designation – Texas
- Texas 10 Step Facility
- Women's Choice Award America's 100 Best Hospitals for Patient Experience (2011-2019)
- Safe Riders Child Safety Seat Distribution and Education Program
- Best Companies to Work for in Texas (8 years)
- American College of Surgeons Commission on Cancer – Three Year Accreditation with Commendation
- Breast Imaging Center of Excellence by ACR
- Computed Tomography Accreditation by ACR
- Breast Ultrasound Accreditation by ACR
- Breast Ultrasound Biopsy Accreditation by ACR
- Echocardiography Accreditation by IAC
- Stereotactic Breast Biopsy Accreditation by ACR
- Vascular Ultrasound Accreditation by ACR
- College of American Pathologist Accredited Laboratory
- Texas Department of State Health Services - Primary Level II Stroke Facility
- Level III NICU Designation
- International Board-Certified Lactation Consultant (IBCLC) Care Award

CHRISTUS St. Michael Rehabilitation Hospital

- Texarkana Gazette Best Physical Therapy/Rehab (2019)
- Named as one of the industry's best rehabilitation facilities by Rehab Management (2011, 2012, 2013)
- CARF Accredited Inpatient Rehabilitation Program & Stroke Specialty Program
- The Joint Commission Accredited
- Texas Award for Performance Excellence (all facilities and HH surveyed) (2014)
- Press Ganey Guardian of Excellence Award (2015, 2016)

CSM-Atlanta

- American College of Cardiology Accreditation-Chest Pain Center Accreditation
- AHA/ASA Target: Stroke Honor Roll-Elite– Silver Plus Award Quality Achievement (2019)
- Accredited by The Joint Commission
- Texas Award for Performance Excellence (all facilities and HH surveyed) (2014)
- College of American Pathologists Accredited Laboratory
- Level IV Trauma Center Designation in the State of Texas
- Press Ganey Guardian of Excellence Award (2015)

-       Texas Department of State Health Services - Level III Stroke Facility

Services/Programs Unique to CHRISTUS St. Michael Health System

Cardiology Services
-       Region's only Electrophysiology Lab – full-service compliment including mapping and ablation procedures
-       Region's only Open-Heart Surgery Program

Imaging Services
-       Breast Imaging Center of Excellence
-       Accredited CT Cardiac/Coronary Imaging
-       Stereotactic Breast Biopsy Accreditation by ACR

Oncology Services
-       Bio Banking Research/Clinical Trials (blood and tissue studies)
-       Cancer Survivorship Program
-       Genetic Counseling & Testing with Certified Cancer Genetic Educator
-       Cancer Center RN Triage Call Line
-       Cancer Services Symptom Management Clinic
-       High Dose Radiation for lung, gynecological cancer

- Immunotherapy
- In-house, full-time Medical Physicist
- Two Oncology Social workers
- Outpatient Oncology Rehabilitation
- Palliative Care Clinic
- Prone Breast Radio Therapy
- Savi Breast Brachy Therapy
- TruBeam Linear Accelerator

Other Services
- Center for Joint Replacement
- Joint Commission Disease-Specific Certification for Hip and Knee
- Joint Commission Disease-Specific Certification for Spine Surgery
- Outpatient Infusion Therapy 7 days a week
- Outpatient Pulmonary Rehabilitation
- Medically-Based Health & Fitness Center

Inpatient Rehabilitation
- CARF Certified Inpatient Rehabilitation Hospital

Outpatient Rehabilitation
- Balance Rehabilitation
- Biodex Testing
- Blood Flow Restriction Therapy
- Certified Dry Needling

- Certified Hand Therapy
- Certified Lymphedema Therapy
- Certified Manual Therapy
- Certified Sports Specialization
- Driving Evaluation
- Functional Capacity Evaluation/Physical Performance Testing
- Nerve Conduction Velocity Testing
- Post-Offer Employment Testing
- Power Wheelchair Evaluations

Women and Children's
- Neonatal Intensive Care Unit (babies as young as 23 weeks gestation)
- Continuing Care Nursery

Surgical Services
- Hybrid Surgical Suite
- Two (2) da Vinci Surgical Robots
- Robotic-Assisted Total Knee Replacement
- ERAS (Enhanced Recovery After Surgery)
- Strong for Surgery

Appendix B

Annual Report to the Bishop Joseph Strickland

Diocese of Tyler, Texas

Reproduced with the permission of CHRISTUS St. Michael Health System

Annual Report of Activity

Prepared for Bishop Joseph Strickland,

Diocese of Tyler, Texas

CHRISTUS St. Michael Health System review of the activities undertaken in Fiscal Year 2016 to support our Catholic Health Care Ministry. Our Mission: "to extend the healing ministry of Jesus Christ."

6/30/2016

Report for the Bishop
Diocese of Tyler, Texas
Activity Fiscal Year
Submitted on behalf of CHRISTUS St. Michael
Health System
June 30, 2016

OUR MISSION: *To Extend the Healing Ministry of Jesus Christ* "

CHRISTUS®
ST. MICHAEL HEALTH SYSTEM

June 30, 2016

Most Reverend Joseph E. Strickland
Bishop of Tyler
1015 ESE Loop 323
Tyler, TX 75701-9663

Your Excellency:

CHRISTUS St. Michael Health System is appreciative of all your support for our Ministry. It is our honor to be partners with the Diocese in sponsoring the Parish Nursing Program in cooperation with Catholic Charities East Texas.

It is our desire to expand this program as well as look for other ways to partner with the Diocese to spread the word of Jesus' love.

I have attached a report of CHRISTUS St. Michael's activities in support of our Mission for Fiscal Year 2016. Sr. Jean Connell, Chris Karam, and I would like to arrange a time to come to Tyler to discuss our Ministry with you. We want to look at other opportunities to work together in ways that improve the well-being of our residents, strengthens our relationship with the local churches in the Diocese, and, most importantly, reinforces our Identity as a Ministry of the Catholic Church with our Associates and physicians.

I will work with your assistant to arrange a convenient time to meet before July 1 this year.

Again, thank you for your support of our Ministry.

Respectfully yours,
Fr. Lawrence Chellaian
Vice President, Mission Integration

Introduction: CHRISTUS St. Michael Health System has continued to use CATHOLIC IDENTITY MATRIX (CIM) as the foundational instrument for assessing our fidelity to acting as Ministry of the Catholic Church and consistency with our Mission Statement *"to extend the Healing Ministry of Jesus Christ."*

The enclosed report is a brief overview of the Health System's activities during the fiscal year 2016. The report uses the principles outlined in the CIM as the basis for providing information.

Solidarity with the Poor: CHRISTUS St. Michael Health System takes the approach that Solidary with the Poor consists of more than the provision of charity care. Our way of showing our solidary includes activities that will improve access to care. We believe access to primary care and increased health literacy among our service area residents are critical components of our solidarity with those in poverty. As a result, we have engaged the community in the following activities:

- Acting as the leader in the expansion of the Federally Qualified Health Center (Genesis PrimeCare) within the Texarkana location. The Center provides adult and pediatric primary care, obstetrical dental health, and mental health services. In

January 2016, the services were expanded to include a location in Texarkana, Arkansas. The addition of this location allowed low-income residents from that part of the service area also to access affordable primary care. All services are provided in a manner consistent with the Ethical and
Religious Directives for Catholic Health Care Services.

- Transitional nursing services funded by Delivery
System Reform Incentive Payments (DSRIP) in cooperation with UT Tyler to help patients avoid
hospitalization has expanded and successfully met
or exceeded all project goals. This result will allow
the program to continue to be funded through
DSRIP.

- The Advance Care planning program, which allows
individuals to have a say in the medical decisions
that affect their lives, has been expanded with additional emphasis placed on helping patients in Palliative Care have access to assistance in creating a
plan.

- Financially sponsor a Parish Nurse network in collaboration with Catholic Charities East Texas, including 8 churches in Texarkana. The congregations involved include mainline protestant and
non-denominational churches that have older and

diverse congregations. All churches involve in the
Network have signed agreements assuring all services provided as part of the Parish Nurse Network
with be consistent with the Ethical and Religious
Directives for Catholic Health Care Services.

- CHRISTUS St. Michael's administration was the
  main driving force in assuring that the Mental
  Health Regional Crisis Center was established in
  CSM-Atlanta. The Crisis Center has admitted 587
  patients in the fiscal year, with only 12% requiring
  readmission. The program allows persons who
  have a mental illness to be directed to ongoing
  supportive care after their inpatient stay.

- CHRISTUS St. Michael, with the support of
  CHRISTUS Health, led the Affordable Care Act
  enrollment effort for our service area. The project
  enrolled 4502 Bowie County, Texas, and Miller
  County, Arkansas residents into health insurance
  programs. CHRISTUS St. Michael also join forces
  with the Ark-Tex Council of governments to create
  a premium support program that assisted 226 Texas residents who had incomes of between 100%
  and 150% of the federal poverty guideline to pay
  their health insurance premium. This program is
  unique and may be the only one of its type initiated
  by a Catholic health care organization.

- Completed the third year of operation of Downtown Community Garden started by the Downtown Texarkana Clergy Alliance started with the financial support of CHRISTUS St. Michael Health System. Two and one-half (2.5) tons have been harvested and distributed to local poverty agencies during the fiscal year.

- Assisted organizations in securing funding through the CHRISTUS Fund. This fiscal year we were successful in gaining renewal of Parish Nurse funding in conjunction with Catholic Charities East Texas and funding for CASA of a medical screening service for children who are victims of sexual abuse. Assisted local community agencies in securing funding from the CHRISTUS Fund. The most recent award was to Catholic Charities East Texas for the continuation of the Parish Nurse program.

- Associates and the organization were financial supporters as well as volunteers for Cancer Society, American Heart Association, WJ Running Ranch, Temple Rehabilitation, Community Healthcore, Clay Eichler Foundation, Hospice of Texarkana, Alzheimer's Alliance, Bishop of Tyler Annual Appeal, CASA, Harvest Texarkana, Downtown Ministerial Alliance Community Garden, Randy Sam's Shelter, Salvation Army, Grace

Free Medical Clinic, St. Edwards Catholic Outreach Center, Liberty-Eylau Foundation, Habitat for Humanity, Texarkana College, Hospice of Texarkana and Texarkana Nursing Advisory Board. Community Benefit contributions and grants equaled $596,000 in addition to the volunteer time of our Associates and leaders.

- The organization and its Associates were the second largest contributor to the annual United Way Campaign.

- We provided $19.3 million in Charity Care.

- Sponsor the Spirit of St. Michael van to do immunization, general health status, and asthma screening

- Funded the Health Teacher/Go Noodle project providing an integrated health curriculum to 63 elementary schools with 22,000 students participating in our primary service area

- Active in providing mentors to "at-risk" children in the Texarkana Texas School district.

- Residence training of Family Practice Doctors for AHEC

- Training site for Texarkana College, University of Arkansas Community College, and South Arkansas Community College for Allied Health Professionals training.

- Simulation Lab training for health care professionals with an emphasis on Skilled Nursing staff.
- "iPad" project to assist in reducing readmissions.

Participatory Workplace: Within CHRISTUS St. Michael, we use the Principle of Subsidiarity. This tenet holds that nothing should be done by a larger and more complex organization, which can be done as well by a smaller and simpler organization. In other words, any activity which a more decentralized entity can perform should be. Using this principle as a basis for decision-making CHRISTUS St. Michael has 'hardwired" a process of ethical decision-making labeled Values-Based Decision Making.

CHRISTUS St. Michael Boards and Senior Leadership often are called upon to make critical decisions concerning strategic planning and operational issues. These issues touch the core of our Catholic Identity. These decisions impact both the communities we serve and our Associates. The Ministry of CHRISTUS St. Michael is rooted in faith and guided by Catholic Health Care values. In the current environment, health care often is viewed as an industry or business. Therefore, it is more imperative than ever that our faith-based health system's decisions are grounded in the faith and values that CHRISTUS St. Michael strives to embody. The Values-Based Decision-Making Process is intended to provide a mechanism to discuss and clarify the mission/ethical dimensions of major proposals and initiatives. The process serves as the operational link, which facilitates the integration of the mission/ values/vision/ethical perspectives into these decisions. CHRISTUS St. Michael also uses these additional tactics to increase communication and support a collaborative workplace:

- **Associate Rounding** - This consists of leaders rounding with Associates to allow leaders to answer any tough questions that any Associate may have. Rounding strengthens communication and recognizes Associates as experts for recognizing others, improving processes and safety.

- **Daily Patient Care Rounding**- Our Chief Medical Officer, Chief of Medical Affairs, Chief Nursing Executive, and Director of Case management do daily rounds on each patient care unit. The Chief Financial Officer and Vice President of Mission Integration also assist in completing rounds regularly. The leaders assist nurses and other caregivers in providing patient-centered care. The focus is on education and assistance in assuring the evidence-based, best practices care is being given to all patients.

- **Town Hall Meetings** - Held quarterly, 16 meetings are held over a period for all shifts, and of those 16, some are held at all CHRISTUS St. Michael locations, so the associates do not have to travel to the acute-care hospital. Our CEO and Regional COO lead these.

- **Cascade Learning** is a behavior that has been implemented in our business philosophy. When our organization leaders participate in our off-site Leadership Development Institute (LDI), the new skills and tools they learned at the institute are cascaded to all associates within one month of returning from LDI. This practice is an opportunity for our leaders to share what they learned and allows our Associates to ask questions about the new learning.

- **KUDOS** - Online Recognition Program rewards and recognizes Associates through the KUDOS Program to promote and provide excellent service and exemplify CHRISTUS core values.

- **Quarterly Incentive celebrations & payouts** - all associates are eligible for this incentive payout. These awards are based on meeting or exceeding our aligned organizational goals.

- **Success Factors**- An Associate supervisor method of creating goals in a collaborative manner

- **Best Place to Work-** CHRISTUS St. Michael was chosen as the best place to work in Texarkana for the sixth consecutive year and one of the best places to work in Texas for the eighth year. Eighty- percent (80%) of Associates in the Associate Satisfaction survey say being a faith-based organization is their principal reason for working at the Health Center.

CHRISTUS St. Michael was also recertified as a "Magnet" Hospital for Nursing Services. A Magnet-designated hospital is an organization that has been recognized by the American Nurses Credentialing Center (ANCC) after demonstrating excellence in patient care in more than 35 areas of focus throughout the entire hospital. The Magnet Recognition Program® provides the ultimate benchmark for patients and their families to measure the quality of care they can expect at a hospital. It is called "Magnet" because of the ability to attract and retain professional nurses. One of our nursing organizational design's critical characteristics is the Nursing Councils for each service provided.

Holistic Care: CHRISTUS St. Michael continues to implement the plan of Physician Formation first begun in 2016. This plan includes:

- Invitation to physicians to lunch with Chaplains to have an opportunity to discuss the interaction of spiritual and physical needs.
- Conducting an Ethics and Catholic Health Care 4-hour intensive workshop attended by 34 providers in November 2015. It is planned to have an annual

intensive workshop with CME credit to reinforce the Mission Driven purpose of our work

- We have expanded the Palliative Care Program to include a multidisciplinary team approach with a Palliative Care Physician, Advanced Practice Nurses, RN, Social work, Pharmacy, and Spiritual Care. We are now seeing an average of nearly 100 physicians who requested consultations each month.

- They have been increased meeting with the Ethics consultation team that is led by two Certified Medical bioethicists. In June 2016, a two-day intensive training program was conducted to train five additional staff members to be able to conduct Clinical Ethics consultations.

- We have increased the active participation of physicians on the Ethics Committee.

- We have designed training for aligned (primarily employed) physicians, including hospitalists, intensivists, ED, and resident doctors, concerning the importance of "doing for as opposed to doing to" patients.

- We mandate the orientation of every physician who is new to the medical staff. The orientation is conducted by the Vice President of Mission Integration or the Director of Spiritual Care. This same training is provided to all aligned physicians, including specialists. The orientation is focused explicitly on ensuring all physicians understand our Catholic Ministry and Mission.

- We offer continuous education and opportunities to invite clinical and support staff to be affirmed for actions that reinforce our Mission and Values. The "Kudos" program has proved to be an extraordinarily successful tool in affirming Associates.

- As noted in the preceding section, we have instituted a program of daily rounding on all units. The rounding team includes the Chief Medical Officers, Chief Nursing Officer, Director of Case Management, Chief Financial officer, and the Mission Leader. Patient care plans are reviewed with attending nurses and case management staff daily to ensure they have the resources they need.

Respect for Life: Several years ago, CHRISTUS St. Michael decided in consultation with the Bishop of the Diocese of Tyler to discontinue elective sterilizations. During 2016 we added three (3) Obstetricians to our medical staff to augment our existing staff of six (6) physicians. We continue to operate in a manner that is consistent with the ERDs. Moreover, we were given the distinction of a Center of Excellence for Women's Services for the fifth consecutive year. According to independent surveys done by local and national organizations, we are the health care facility of choice for women in our service area. The number one reason that families choose CHRISTUS to have their babies is reported to be "the faith-based way we serve our patients."

CHRISTUS St. Michael has had nurses who have done assessments of patients concerning appropriateness for Palliative Care Services. This service was under a contractual arrangement with a local hospice provider. In 2016 we discontinued the contract. We have created a Palliative Care Team, which would include a Physician, Advanced Practice Nurse, Social worker, Chaplain, and consultation from two pharmacists we now have in training to be Palliative Care Certified. The program is a model within the CHRISTUS Health System to transition patients to appropriate levels of care and confidence shown by attending physicians, as evidenced by the high volume of physician directed consultations.

Stewardship: CHRISTUS St. Michael initiated a Strategic Planning process in Fiscal Year 2016, which identifies the critical strategic goals for the organization. I have attached the one-page summary that demonstrates an understanding of managing the "Mission/Margin" balance that is required to maintain a sustainable ministry.

As part of CHRISTUS Health, we also closely monitor what we call "Compass 20/20. COMPASS 2020 demonstrates a commitment to excellence by focusing on a few key destination points and critical pathways. Key destination points of clinical integration, asset growth, and building a culture of diversity.

During the calendar and fiscal year 2016, CHRISTUS St. Michael achieved or exceeded nearly all expectations for performance in compass 20/20.

Acts in Communion with the Church: The Vice President for Mission Integration is explicitly responsible for the following duties:

1. Assuring that all Policies, Procedures, and Practices of the organization are consistent with the Catholic Church's teachings and are expressly acknowledged in all written policy statements. Each policy, be it clinical, financial, or quality, has an express statement in the Preamble that identifies the Principle of Catholic Health Care, Value, or relationship to the Mission. The Mission Leader is a member of the Administrative team who is involved with all aspects of the operation, including the development of relationships with non-Catholic entities, mergers, and acquisitions that are being contemplated. As a member of the Administrative Team, the Mission

leader is also involved in leading the Values-Based Decision-Making process within leadership.

2. The Mission Leader is also responsible for assuring that Spiritual Care Services are conducted through a staffing model that provides qualified chaplains 24 hours/ 7 days per week. Additionally, the Mission Leader **is** responsible for working with the Director of Spiritual Care Services to assure ongoing formation programs are available to all Associates. CHRISTUS St. Michael utilizes the Leadership Development Institute for all managers and directors as an ongoing venue for providing spiritual formation experiences. These events are held quarterly. We also sponsor regular monthly meetings with physicians to discuss the integration of spiritual and physical care.

   CHRISTUS St. Michael Board Members were invited to participate in an annual planning retreat in which there is a focus on the integration of the Mission with the execution of the business plan. The event was held in June 2016 with nearly all board members present in addition to planning staff from the System office. The session's focus was planning for a future in which Catholic health care will be severely challenged to maintain focus on Mission while being prudent stewards of the gifts given to us by our Creator.

3. The Mission leader is responsible for Organization and Clinical Ethics. The organization has an active Ethics committee that meets six times per year. The Ethics committee has representation from all aligned physician groups, Palliative Care, all clinical nursing areas, the CEO, CNE, and CMO. The committee has several subcommittees, including:

- Patient Right
- Organizational/business ethics
- Advance Care planning
- Policy Review
- Ethics Consultation Team.

The Ethics consultation team is made up of 2 Certified Medical Bioethicists, a physician, and the Mission Leader who have both been provided training through the National Catholic Bioethics Center. Ethics Consultation requests are responded to with 24-hours. In 2016 there were 32 documented Ethics consultations with all situations being resolved to the clinicians' and families' satisfaction. In June 2016, we trained an additional five (5) members of the staff, which included two (2) physicians and three (3) Registered Nurses, to be members of the clinical ethics team to assure we could respond to requests in a timely basis.

4. **Community Benefit**: CHRISTUS St. Michael provides over 13% of its operating expense for charity and community benefit. Community Benefit includes such includes physician, nurse, and allied health professional education. Partnership with the Federally Qualified Health Center, local school districts, community mental health, homeless services, and the "Spirit of St. Michael" mobile medical clinic. We also worked in conjunction with Catholic Charities East Texas to establish a Parish Nursing Network in Texarkana. The Health Center also led the community effort to enroll persons in the Health Care Exchange and the Private Option health insurance plans.

   Employee Assistance Program: CHRISTUS St. Michael provides an "in-house" counseling service that provides mental health, chemical dependency, and family assistance. The program also sponsors a health and financial awareness program. The Health Center also provides no-interest loans to associates with short-term acute financial needs. This activity serves over 100 Associates in 2016 and kept them from depending on "payday" loans. All associates receiving loans are also enrolled in a financial counseling service to assist them in "money management."

Conclusion: CHRISTUS St. Michael Health System is committed to assuring that we can demonstrate our fidelity to the Mission we have stated in a way that is both quality and quantifiably able to be measured. We believe that if we do not intentionally evaluate our Catholic Identity as a foundational element of our purpose that we will be deluded into believing "good works" is enough. We believe that our actions must be representative of our faithfulness to the Mission of "extending the healing ministry of Jesus Christ.

Appendix C

Catholic Identity Matrix

Executive Summary Submitted to CHRISTUS ST. Michael Health System, June 24, 2013, by the Veritas Institute, Opus College of Business, University of St. Thomas, St. Paul, Minnesota

Establishing and sustaining institutional identity is a significant challenge for leaders in Catholic health care. The Catholic Identity Matrix (CIM) enables a Catholic health care institution to gain a realistic, evidence-based understanding of how well it has embedded six principles for Catholic health care within its management system. These principles are Solidarity with those who live in poverty, holistic care, respect for human life, participatory community of work and mutual respect, stewardship, and acting in communion with the Church.

A CIM assessment was conducted at CHRISTUS St. Michael Health System of Texarkana, TX, on April 25, 2013. The assessment provides a qualitative and quantitative portrait of the extent to which the six principles for

Catholic health care have been integrated within CHRISTUS St. Michael's operating policies and processes. The CIM's results also identify opportunities to better institutionalize these principles within the hospital's management system and establish a baseline from which future improvements may be gauged.

The results of the CIM assessment underscore two overarching strengths. First, the assessment teams' comments suggest that CHRISTUS St. Michael's leaders and associates are strongly committed to its mission and identity as a Catholic health care institution. Second, CHRISTUS St. Michael's efforts to embed the six principles for Catholic health care within its management system are comprehensive and mature. The institution's activities address the CIM assessment matrix's full scope, while scores for 35 of the 36 cells within the matrix fell in Category 4, 5, or 6, the top three performance classifications. These scores are among the highest recorded to date in a CIM application. They indicate an institution that has developed the capacity to systematically support Catholic health care's six principles. Furthermore, these scores suggest that the organization's efforts have been largely consistent across the six principles. In short, CHRISTUS St. Michael has established a comprehensive and capable foundation for systematically advancing its mission as a Catholic health care ministry.

That said, there remain opportunities for CHRISTUS St. Michael to institutionalize its Catholic identity more fully. Among these, the following are notable:

- Integrating explicit references within policies and processes to CHRISTUS St. Michael's foundational moral convictions - as represented, for example, by its Core Values, the *Ethical and Religious Directives for Catholic Health Care Services,* or the six principles for Catholic health care principles - to help associates understand more readily how the institution's Catholic identity animates its operations;

- Enhancing physician alignment with the principles for Catholic health care through educational initiatives (e.g., advanced ERD training, the organization's emerging physician formation program) and by ensuring that aspirations related to these principles are integrated within processes that shape physician relations (e.g., processes for privilege-granting, for selecting contracted physicians, orientation and onboarding practices, performance assessment criteria and review processes, communications, etc.);

- Creating interview guidelines or questions linked to critical elements of the CHRISTUS St. Michael's Catholic identity and applying them consistently within interviews for senior roles to ensure a commitment to these principles is sustained within the organization's leadership;

- Documenting informal practices that have emerged over time to support Solidarity with the poor and acting in communion with the Church, to integrate them more formally within operations and promote their continuous improvement;

- Enhancing the religious diversity present among CHRISTUS St. Michael's chaplains to better match the range of faith perspectives present within the population the organization serves;

- Strengthening current efforts to act as a good steward of the natural environment and natural resources;

- Broadening collaborations within the local community to more effectively address the needs of the poor and the marginalized; and

- Examining the process CHRISTUS St. Michael uses to enhance its training offerings to ensure this approach is both capable and utilized regularly.

Index

Scriptural References

Scripture	Page	Scripture	Page
Gn 1:1-31	52	1 Kgs 19:11	174
Gn 1:26-27	41	1 Kgs 19:12	174-75
Gn 1:27	39	1 Kgs 19:9	175
Gn 1:31	22, 47, 52	2 Kgs 1-2	173
Gn 2:1-3	52	2 Kgs 4: 32-35	89
Gn 2:4-3:24	45-7	2 Kgs 4: 42-43	143
Gn 2:7	46, 49, 62, 83	2 Kgs 4:42-44	89
Gn 3:17-19	48	2 Kgs 4:44	143
Gn 3:19	62	2 Mc 12:40	93
Gn 4:41	88	2 Mc 12:40-45	93
Gn 22:2	87	2 Mc 12:43-46	93
Gn 37:3	88	Jb 3:11-13	79
Gn 37:4	88	Jb 3:14-15a	79
Gn 37:7-10	88	Jb 3:17-19	79
Gn 37:18-20	88	Jb 7: 9-10	80
Gn 37:21-27	88	Jb 10:21	73
Gn 39:7-13	88	Jb 10:21-22	73
Ex 16:1-36	143	Jb 14:7-9	79
Ex 20:1-17	111	Jb 14:13-17	78, 80
Lev 19:9-18	vii	Jb 14:19	79
Lev 19:18	29	Jb 17:13	73
Dt 6:4-5	vii	Jb 17:13-16	73
Dt 6:5	29	Jb 19: 25-27	72-3, 80
Dt 30:6	72	Jb 26:5	73
2 Sm 11:2-4	176	Ps 6:5	73
1 Kgs 1:5-8	177	Ps 16:10	84
1 Kgs 17:21-22	89	Ps 23:4	61
1 Kgs 17:24	173	Ps: 30:2-4	84
1 Kgs 17-19	173	Ps 30:9	73
1 Kgs 18:36	174	Ps 30:12	84
1 Kgs 19:10	174	Ps 37:37-40	85

Ps 49: 14-16	85	Wis 10:3	100
Ps 61:2-5	86	Wis 10:9-14	100
Ps 86:11-13	86	Is 2:4	91
Ps 88:3-5	73	Is 5:14	73
Ps 88:6	73	Is 6:11	91
Ps 88:10-12	73	Is 7:14	92
Ps 94:17	73	Is 9:6	91
Ps 102:5	102	Is 11:1	90
Ps 115:17	73	Is 11:6	91
Ps 139:8	73, 86	Is 11:10	90
Ps 143:3	73	Is 14:9-10	73
Prv 1:12	73	Is 29:17-24	180
Prv 27:20	73	Is 35:5-10	180
Prv 31:26	177	Is 38:10	73
Prv 31:28	177	Is 38:11	73
Prv 31:29	178	Is 38:18	73
Eccl 1:14-18	83	Is 40:3	91
Eccl 9:5	73	Is 42:1-9	90
Eccl 9:6	73	Is 42:6	91
Eccl 9:10	73	Is 49:1-7	90
Eccl 11:7-12	72, 83	Is 49: 6	89
Wis 1:10	97	Is 50:4-11	90
Wis 1:15	94	Is 52:13-53:12	90
Wis 1:15-16	98	Is 53:3	91
Wis 1:16	94-5	Is 65:17	91
Wis 2:2	95	Jer 1:5	114
Wis 2:3	72, 99	Jer 31:31	72
Wis 2:7	99	Bar 2:27-35	72
Wis 2:10	95	Bar 3:4	72
Wis 2:11	95, 99	Ez 3:15	75
Wis 2:12-20	96	Ez 28:11-19	139
Wis 3:7	96	Ez 36:26	xv
Wis 6:17-20	97	Ez 37:1-14	72, 75-6
Wis 6:20	99	Dn 12:1-3	72, 82
Wis 7:26-30	99	Dn 12:2	81, 94

Lk 1:38-42	178	Jn 2:11	151
Lk 1:52	179	Jn 2:18	151
Lk 3:9	123	Jn 2:23	151
Lk 4:1-13	88	Jn 3:16	87
Lk 4:16.30	27	Jn 4:46-54	137
Lk 4:40	24	Jn 5:13	189
Lk 6:20-26	102, 164	Jn 5:19-30	122
LK 7:1-10	137	Jn 5:22-23	122
Lk 8:15	28	Jn 5:27-30	122
Lk 8:22-25	136	Jn 6:1-14	89, 141
Lk 8:26-39	138	Jn 6:3	89
Lk 8:43	147	Jn 6:5-15	143
Lk 9:1-2	226	Jn 6:10	145
Lk 9:12-17	89, 143	Jn 6:16-21	135
Lk 9:27	123	Jn 6:44	164
Lk 9:43-45	122	Jn 6:69	xvii
Lk 10:25-37	227, 228	Jn 8:12	90
Lk 10:36-37	230	Jn 8:27-30	122
Lk 11:50	123	Jn 9:1	147
Lk 13:32	151	Jn 11:1-45	78
Lk 17:5-6	28	Jn 11:43-44	138
Lk 17: 21	28	Jn 12:7-8	122
Lk 18:31-34	122	Jn 12:18	151
Lk 21:32	123	Jn 12:23	122
Lk 22:33-34	88	Jn 12:37	151
Lk 22:39-23:56	88	Jn 13:36-38	88
Lk 22:51	145	Jn 14:26-31	122
Lk 22:50-51	147	Jn 18:1–19:42	88
Lk 24:31	118	Jn 20:14-15	118
Lk 24:50-53	88	Jn 20:17	88
Jn 1:14	91	Jn 20:27	145
Jn 2:1-11	141	Jn 22-23	122
Jn 2:4	142	Acts 1:1-12	88
Jn 2:5	178	Acts 2:22	151
Jn 2:9	145	Acts 3:7	145

Bibliography

Admin. "Conscience, Newman, and The Pope." *The Catholic Thing*, September 18, 2015. https://www.thecatholicthing.org/2015/02/25/conscience-newman-pope/.

Aquinas, Thomas. "Question 23. How the Passions Differ from One Another." *Summa Theologiae* (Prima Secundae Partis, Q. 23), 2017. http://www.newadvent.org/summa/2023.htm.

_. "Question 92. The Vision of the Divine Essence in Reference to the Blessed." *Summa Theologiae* (Supplementum, Q. 92). Accessed February 20, 2021. https://www.newadvent.org/summa/5092.htm.

_. "St. Thomas Aquinas – Summa Contra Gentiles - Book III (Q. 1-83)." *Genius*. Genius Media Group. Accessed February 24, 2021. https://genius.com/St-thomas-aquinas-summa-contra-gentiles-book-iii-q-1-83-annotated.

———. Whether the Passions of the Concupiscible Part are Different from those of the Irascible Part? Bible Hub. Accessed February 24, 2021. https://biblehub.com/library/aquinas/summa_theologica/whether_the_passions_of_the.htm.

Arbuckle, Gerald Anthony. *Catholic Identity or Identities? Refounding Ministries in Chaotic Times*. Collegeville, MN: Liturgical Press, 2013.

Arbuckle, Gerald. "Retelling 'The Good Samaritan.'" *Catholic Health Association*, 2007.

https://www.chausa.org/publications/health-
progress/article/july-august-2007/retelling-the-good-
samaritan-.

Armstrong, Karen. *St. Paul: The Apostle We Love to Hate.* Boston, MA: New Harvest, Houghton Mifflin Harcourt, 2015.

Ascension Health and Veritas Institute of the University of St.
Thomas. *The Catholic Identity Matrix: General Information.*
St. Paul, MN: Veritas Institute, 2020.

Becker, Ernest. *The Denial of Death.* New York: Free Press Paperbacks, 1997.

"Beliefs of World Religions About Origins." *Religious Tolerance.*
Accessed August 10, 2020.
http://www.religioustolerance.org/ev_denom2.htm.

Benedict XVI, Pope. *Dei Verbum.* Accessed February 20, 2021.
http://www.vatican.va/archive/hist_councils/ii_vatican_coun
cil/documents/vat-ii_const_19651118_dei-verbum_lt.html.

Benedict XVI, Pope. *Verbum Domini*: Post-Synodal Apostolic
Exhortation on the Word of God in the Life and Mission of
the Church (30 September 2010) | BENEDICT XVI. Libreria
Editrice Vaticana, September 29, 2010.
http://www.vatican.va/content/benedict-
xvi/en/apost_exhortations/documents/hf_ben-
xvi_exh_20100930_verbum-domini.html.

Bergsma, John Sietze, and Brant James Pitre. *A Catholic Introduction to the Bible.* 1. Vol. 1. San Francisco: Ignatius Press,
2018.

Boyett, Jason. *12 Major World Religions: The Beliefs, Rituals, and
Traditions of Humanity's Most Influential Faiths.* Berkeley,
CA: Zephyros Press, 2016.

Bratcher, Dennis. "The 'Fall' - A Second Look A Literary Analy-
    sis of Genesis 2:4-3:24." The Fall - A Second Look: Genesis 3.
    Accessed January 18, 2020.
    http://www.crivoice.org/gen3.html.

Casey, Juliana M. *Food for the Journey: Theological Foundations
    of the Catholic Healthcare Ministry.* St. Louis, MO: Catholic
    Health Association of the United States, 1991.

*Catechism of the Catholic Church: with Modifications from the
    Editio Typica.* New York: Doubleday, 2003.

"Catholic Health Care in America." Facts - Statistics." *Catholic
    Health Association,* January 2020.
    https://www.chausa.org/about/about/facts-statistics.

Clark, David. "From Margins to Centre: A Review of the
    History of Palliative Care in Cancer." *Lancet Oncology*
    8, no. 5 (May 2007): 430–38.
    https://doi.org/https://doi.org/10.1016/S1470-
    2045(07)70138-9.

_. "Palliative Medicine as a Specialty." End of Life Studies.
    University   of   Glasgow,   October   4,   2016.
    http://endoflifestudies.academicblogs.co.uk/palliative-
    medicine-as-a-specialty

Coggins, R. "Job." Essay. In *The Oxford Bible Commentary,* edit-
    ed by John Barton and John Muddiman, 433–84. Oxford:
    Oxford University Press, 2007.

Committee on Approaching Death: Addressing Key End of Life
    Issues. "The Delivery of Person-Centered, Family-Oriented
    End-of-Life Care." *Dying in America: Improving Quality and
    Honoring Individual Preferences Near the End of Life.* U.S.

National Library of Medicine, March 19, 2015. https://www.ncbi.nlm.nih.gov/books/NBK285676/.

Coulter-Harris, Deborah M. *Chasing Immortality in World Religions.* Jefferson, North Carolina: McFarland & Company, Inc., 2016.

Dault, Kira. "What Is the Preferential Option for the Poor?" *U.S. Catholic.* U.S. Catholic Magazine, January 2015. http://www.uscatholic.org/articles/201501/what-preferential-option-poor-29649.

Dauphinais, Michael, and Matthew Levering. *Holy People, Holy Land: A Theological Introduction to the Bible.* Grand Rapids, MI: Brazos Press, 2005.

"Defining the Medical Home." *Patient-Centered Primary Care Collaborative.* January 17, 2019. https://www.pcpcc.org/about/medical-home.

Dunning, H. Ray, and Neil B. Wiseman. *Biblical Resources for Holiness Preaching: from Text to Sermon.* Kansas City, MO: Beacon Hill Press, 1990.

Esposito, John L. *The Islam the Straight Path.* New York: Oxford University Press, 2016.

Ethical and Religious Directives for Catholic Health Care Services. Washington, D.C., DC: United States Conference of Catholic Bishops, 2018.

Fisher, George P. *Manual of Christian Evidences.* New York: Charles Scribner's Sons, 1894.

Francis, Francine, and Stacey Magness. *100 Years of Healing: CHRISTUS St. Michael.* Texarkana, Texas: CHRISTUS St. Michael Health System, September 2016.

Fuller, Reginald H., and Daniel Alfred Westberg. *Preaching the Lectionary: The Word of God for the Church Today.* Collegeville, MN: Liturgical Press, 2006.

Greenleaf, Robert K. *Servant Leadership: A Journey into the Nature of Legitimate Power and Greatness.* Edited by Larry C. Spears. Mahwah, NJ: Paulist Press, 2002.

"Half of US Catholic Hospitals Do Sterilizations, Report Suggests: News Headlines." *Catholic World News*, February 12, 2012. https://www.catholicculture.org/news/headlines/index.cfm?storyid=13400.

Hammes, Bud. "History of Respecting Choices®." *Respecting Choices.* Accessed January 2, 2020. https://respectingchoices.org/about-us/history-of-respecting-choices/.

Hardon, John A. "Meaning of Virtue in Thomas Aquinas." *EWTN Global Catholic Television Network.* Accessed July 18, 2020. https://www.ewtn.com/catholicism/library/meaning-of-virtue-in-thomas-aquinas-12609.

Hatkoff, Craig, Irwin Kula, and Zach Levine. "How To Die In America: Welcome To La Crosse, Wisconsin." *Forbes Magazine*, October 4, 2014. https://www.forbes.com/sites/offwhitepapers/2014/09/23/how-to-die-in-america-welcome-to-la-crosse/#2d005c0be8c6.

Hooper, Walter. *C.S. Lewis: A Complete Guide to His Life and Works.* San Francisco: HarperSanFrancisco, 1996.

Horbury, William. "The Wisdom of Solomon." Essay. In *The Oxford Bible Commentary*, edited by John Barton and John

Muddiman, 650–67. Oxford, New York: Oxford University Press, 2007.

"In U.S., Decline of Christianity Continues at Rapid Pace." *Pew Research Center's Religion & Public Life Project*, June 9, 2020. https://www.pewforum.org/2019/10/17/in-u-s-decline-of-christianity-continues-at-rapid-pace/.

"Informed Consent." *American Medical Association.* Accessed December 22, 2019. https://www.ama-assn.org/delivering-care/ethics/informed-consent.

"Inpatient Palliative Care Program." *Center to Advance Palliative Care*, February 25, 2019.
https://www.capc.org/toolkits/starting-the-program/designing-an-inpatient-palliative-care-program/.

Jackson, Wayne. "What Does the Bible Say About Miracles?" *Christian Courier*, 2019.
https://www.christiancourier.com/articles/5-what-does-the-bible-say-about-miracles.

Jensen, Steven J. *Living the Good Life: A Beginner's Thomistic Ethics.* Washington, DC: Catholic University of America Press, 2013.

John F. Crosby." The Catholic Thing, September 14, 2019. https://www.thecatholicthing.org/author/jf-crosby/.

Johnson, Luke Timothy. *The Gospel of Luke.* Edited by Daniel J. Harrington. Collegeville, MN: Liturgical Press, 2006.

Johnston, Derek. *A Brief History of Theology: From the New Testament to Feminist Theology.* London: Bloomsbury Publishing PLC, 2008.

jointcommission.org. Accessed June 9, 2020.

https://www.jointcommission.org/accreditation-and-
certification/certification/certifications-by-setting/hospital-
certifications/palliative-care-certification/.

"Joseph, a Type of Christ - Comparison List - Old Testament
Charts." *Bible History Online.* Accessed January 6, 2020.
https://www.bible-history.com/old-testament/types-
joseph.html.

Kelly, Matthew. *The Four Signs of a Dynamic Catholic.* Hebron,
KY: Dynamic Catholic Institute, 2012.

Kierkegaard, Søren. *Fear and Trembling, and: The Sickness unto
Death.* Translated by Walter Lowrie. Princeton, NJ: Princeton University Press, 2013.

Kreeft, Peter J. *A Shorter Summa: The Most Essential Philosophical Passages of St. Thomas Aquinas' Summa Theologica.* San
Francisco: Ignatius Press, 1993.

Kubler-Ross, Elisabeth. *Death and Dying.* New York: Macmillan,
1969.

"Les Provinciales." *Encyclopædia Britannica.* Accessed February
21, 2021. https://www.britannica.com/biography/Blaise-
Pascal/Les-Provinciales#ref365135.

Lewis, C. S. *Miracles: A Preliminary Study.* San Francisco:
HarperOne, 2001.

Lewis, C. S. *The Problem of Pain.* London: HarperCollins, 2002.

Long, Jeffrey, and Paul Perry. *God and the Afterlife: The Groundbreaking New Evidence for God and Near-Death Experience.*
New York: HarperOne, an imprint of HarperCollins Publishers, 2017.

Lysaught, M. Therese. *Caritas in Communion: Theological Foundations of Catholic Health Care.* St. Louis, MO: Catholic Health Association of the United States, 2014.

MacCulloch, Diarmaid. *Christianity: The First Three Thousand Years.* New York: Penguin Books, 2011.

Marshall, Taylor. *Thomas Aquinas in 50 Pages: A Layman's Quick Guide to Thomism.* Irving, TX: Saint John Press, 2014.

Maylone and Benjamin D. Sommers, Bethany, and Benjamin D. Sommers. "Evidence from the Private Option: The Arkansas Experience." *Commonwealth Fund,* February 22, 2017. https://www.commonwealthfund.org/publications/issue-briefs/2017/feb/evidence-private-option-arkansas-experience.

McCurley, Foster R. *Proclamation Commentaries: The Old Testament Witnesses for Preaching.* Philadelphia: Fortress Press, 1978.

Meister, Chad V., and J. B. Stump. *Christian Thought: A Historical Introduction.* London: Routledge, 2017.

Miller, Robert D. *Understanding the Old Testament: Course Guidebook.* Chantilly, VA: The Great Courses, 2019.

Millgram, Hillel I. *The Elijah Enigma: The Prophet, King Ahab, and the Rebirth of Monotheism in the Book of Kings.* Jefferson, NC: McFarland & Company, Inc., Publishers, 2014.

"Miracle." Catholic Answers, February 22, 2019. https://www.catholic.com/encyclopedia/miracle.org

Moltmann Jürgen. *Ethics of Hope.* Minneapolis, MN: Fortress Press, 2012.

Morris, John D. "Do Muslims Believe in Creation?" *The Institute for Creation Research*, December 10, 1992. https://www.icr /article/do-Muslims-believe-creation/.

Murphy-O'Connor, Jerome. *Paul a Critical Life*. Oxford: Oxford University Press, 2012.

Newman, John Henry. "Letter to the Duke of Norfolk, Chapter 5." Accessed December 14, 2019. http://www.newmanreader.org/works/anglicans/volume2/gl adstone/section5.html.

Nichols, Aidan. *The Shape of Catholic Theology: An Introduction to Its Sources, Principles, and History*. Collegeville, MN: The Liturgical Press, 1991.

O'Brien, Dan. "Palliative Care and the Catholic Healing Ministry: Biblical and Historical Roots." Essay. In *Palliative Care and Catholic Health Care: Two Millennia of Caring for the Whole Person*, edited by Peter J. Cataldo and Dan O'Brien, 9–24. Cham, Switzerland: Springer, 2019.

O'Collins, Gerald, and Edward G. Farrugia. *A Concise Dictionary of Theology*. New York: Paulist Press, 2000.

Pally, Marcia. "Theological Resistance." *Commonweal Magazine*, February 14, 2021. https://www.commonwealmagazine.org/theological-resistance.

Panicola, Michael R. *An Introduction to Health Care Ethics: Theological Foundations, Contemporary Issues, and Controversial Cases*. Winona, MN: Anselm Academic, 2007.

Picarello, Anthony R., and Michael F. Moses. "CMS-1625-P." *United States Conference of Catholic Bishops*, September 4, 2015.

http://www.usccb.org/about/general-counsel/rulemaking/upload/Comments-Advance-Directives-Medicare-9-15.pdf.

Pinckaers, Servais Théodore. *Morality: The Catholic View.* Translated by Michael Sherwin. South Bend, IN: St. Augustine's Press, 2001.

Pinker, Aron. "Job's Perspectives on Death." *Jewish Biblical Quarterly* 35, no. 2 (2007): 73–85.

Pius XI, Pope. "Library: Studiorum Ducem (On St. Thomas Aquinas)." *Catholic Culture.* Accessed February 24, 2021. https://www.catholicculture.org/culture/library/view.cfm?rec num=4957.

Pontifical Biblical Commission. "The Interpretation of the Bible in the Church." *Origin*, April 23, 1993. httphttp://www.catholic-resources.org/ChurchDocs/PBC_Interp.htm.

Ratzinger, Joseph. *In the Beginning...The Catholic Understanding of the Story of Creation and the Fall.* Translated by Boniface Ramsey. Grand Rapids, MI: William B Eerdmans Publishing Company, 1995.

Rausch, Thomas P. *Who Is Jesus? An Introduction to Christology.* Collegeville, MN: Liturgical Press, 2003.

Richert, Scott P. "Faith, Hope, and Charity: The Three Theological Virtues for Catholics." *Learn Religions*, January 20, 2019. https://www.learnreligions.com/what-are-the-theological-virtues-542106.

Richter, Karl. "Crossing Guard Hit by Truck in Texarkana to Leave Hospital." *Texarkana Gazette.* November 13, 2020, sec. News.

Robinson, B. A. "Beliefs of World Religions about Origins." *Religious Tolerance.org*. Ontario Consultants on Religious Tolerance, September 15, 2005.
http://www.religioustolerance.org/ev_denom2.htm.

Rolheiser, Ronald. "In Exile." *Saint Louis University Sunday Web Site*. Accessed February 20, 2021.
https://liturgy.slu.edu/EpiphanyB010321/reflections_rolheiser.html.

Sarich, Christina. "Pharma Companies Spend 19x More on Marketing than Research, and Returns Are Dropping." *Natural Society*, May 2, 2017.
http://naturalsociety.com/research-development-new-drugs-not-paying-off-6321/.

Senior, Donald, John J. Collins, and Mary Ann Getty-Sullivan. *The Catholic Study Bible: The New American Bible, Revised Edition*. Third ed. New York: Oxford University Press, 2016.

SGU Pulse. "The Ultimate List of Medical Specialties - Explore Options." *St. George University*, December 11, 2017.
https://www.sgu.edu/blog/medical/ultimate-list-of-medical-specialties/.

Sofield, Loughlan, and Carroll Juliano. *Collaboration: Uniting Our Gifts in Ministry*. Notre Dame, IN, IN: Ave Maria Press, 2000.

Solomon, Sheldon, Jeff Greenberg, and Thomas A. Pyszczynski. *The Worm at the Core: On the Role of Death in Life*. London: Penguin Books, 2016.

Torchia, N. Joseph. "Eschatological Elements in Jesus Healing of the Gerasene Demoniac: An Exegesis of Mk. 5:1--20." *Irish Biblical Studies*, January 2001.

https://biblicalstudies.org.uk/pdf/irish-biblical-studies/23-1_002.pdf.

Trancik, Emily, and Rachelle Barina. "What Makes a Catholic Hospital Catholic?" *U.S. Catholic Magazine,* March 2015. http://www.uscatholic.org/articles/201503/what-makes-catholic-hospital-catholic-29861

US Legal. "Find a Legal Form in Minutes." Emergency Medical Condition Law and Legal Definition. *USLegal, Inc.* Accessed January 20, 2021. https://definitions.uslegal.com/e/emergency-medical-condition

Viviano, Pauline A. *Genesis.* Collegeville, MN: Liturgical Press, 1985.

von Rad, Gerhard. *Genesis. A Commentary.* Translated by John H. P. Marks. London: SCM Press, 1972.

Weinandy, Thomas G. *Does God Suffer?* Notre Dame, IN: Univ. of Notre Dame Press, 2000.

Wenham, David. *Paul: Follower of Jesus or Founder of Christianity?* Grand Rapids: Eerdmans, 1996.

Wills, Garry. *What Paul Meant.* New York: Viking, 2006.

Wrede, William. *The Messianic Secret.* Cambridge: J. Clarke, 1971.

About the Author

The author is a graduate of Southern Illinois University – Edwardsville with a BSW and MA. Mr. Pomeroy later earned his Master of Arts in Health Care Ministry from the Aquinas Institute of Theology in St. Louis, Missouri. He has also recently completed the requirements for a Graduate Certificate in Biblical Studies. He is currently completing the requirements for the Master of Arts in Theology at Aquinas Institute of Theology.

Mr. Pomeroy has been a teacher and social worker. Most notably, he has a career that spans over 40 years as a health care executive with both for-profit and not-for-profit organizations. He recently retired as the Vice President of Mission Integration for CHRISTUS St. Michael Health System.

He has been married to his wife Trudy for 52 years. They have three married children and four grandchildren. They are long-time members of St. Elizabeth Ann Seton Catholic Church in St. Charles, Missouri. Mr. Pomeroy is a 4th Degree Knight of Columbus and in formation to become a Lay Dominican.